Keys to Successfully Living with Your Hearing Loss

Neil G. Bauman, Ph.D.

Integrity First Publications

Stewartstown, PA

http://www.IntegrityFirstPublications.com

Keys to Successfully Living
with Your Hearing Loss

Second Edition

Another **Integrity First** book in the series:

Everything You Wanted to Know About Your Hearing Loss But Were Afraid to Ask
(Because You Knew You Wouldn't Hear the Answers Anyway!)

Copyright 2009, 2011 by Neil G. Bauman

ISBN 978-1-935939-01-6

All rights reserved. No part of this publication may be reproduced or transmitted in any form or by any means, electronic or mechanical, including photocopying, recording or any other information storage and retrieval system without permission in writing from the publisher, except by a reviewer who may quote brief passages in a review.

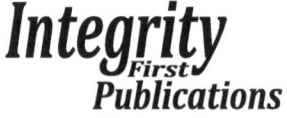

Integrity
First
Publications

49 Piston Court,
Stewartstown, PA 17363-8322
Phone: (717) 993-8555
FAX: (717) 993-6661
Email: info@IntegrityFirstPublications.com
Website: http://www.IntegrityFirstPublications.com

Printed in the United States of America

Contents

About the Author 7

Introduction 9
    Hearing Loss Upsets the Apple Cart! 9
    Six Keys to Successfully Living with Your Hearing Loss 11

**1. The Critical Missing Element to Successfully Living
with Your Hearing Loss—Grieving for Your Hearing Loss** 13
    What Is Grief 14
    The Stages of Grief 15
        Denial 15
        Anger 16
        Bargaining 17
        Depression 17
        Acceptance 18
    The Rest of the Family Needs to Grieve Too 18
    When Is the Right Time to Get Hearing Aids? Where Do Hearing
        Aids Fit into the Grieving Process? 19
    Book to Help You in the Grieving Process 21

**2. Coping with Hearing Loss the Right Way—Why We Act
the Way We Do** 23
    Coping Outcomes 23
    We Often Use Emotion-Focused Rather Than Problem-Focused
        Coping Strategies 24

Example 1: Not Hearing at a Meeting 24
    The Wrong Way 24
    The Right Way 25
Example 2: Bluffing 28
    The Wrong Way 29
    The Right Way 30
Always Think, "Are the Benefits Worthh the Costs?" 32

3. Seven Effective and Free Hearing Loss Coping Strategies 35

1. The Single Most Effective Hearing Loss Coping Strategy—Get Close! 35
   1.1 Sounds Drop Off with Increasing Distance 36
   1.2 Background Noise Becomes a Problem with Increasing Distance 36
   1.3 Speech Becomes Distorted with Increasing Distance 37
   1.4 Speech Intelligence Drops with Increasing Distance 37
   Getting Close—Here's How 38
2. Fair Is- Fair—Go to the Person 38
3. Get the Person's Attention Before Beginning to Talk 39
4. Talk Face-to-Face 39
5. Have Adequate Light 40
6. Cut Out Background Noise 41
7. Avoid Miscommunication—Repeat Back What You Think You Heard—Especially Directions and Instructions 42

4. Hear with Your Eyes—the Art and Science of Speechreading 45

What Is Speechreading? 45
Myths and Realities of Speechreading 47
    Myth 1—All Hard of Hearing People Are Good Speechreaders 47
    Myth 2—You Can Understand Everything When You Speechread 48
Homophenes 48
The Secret to Good Speechreading 49
Speechreading Basics 50
    You Need Reasonable Vision 50
    Always Watch the Person Speaking 50
    Know the Subject and the Context 51
    Slower Is Better 51
    Speechreading Is Tiring 51
    Some People Are Easy to Speechread, Some Aren't 52

5. Hearing Aids—Here's What You Need to Know about Them 55
1. Have the Proper Expectations of What Hearing Aids Can and Cannot Do for You 56
2. How Many Hearing Aids Do You Need? 57
3. Becoming Friends with Your New Hearing Aids 58
4. Which Hearing Aid Is the Best? 59
5. A Dozen Tips to Help You When Buying New Hearing Aids 60

6. Assistive Technology—Turn Your Hearing Aids into Awesome Hearing Devices 65
Benefits of Assistive Listening Devices 66
    You Get Unbelievable Clarity 66
    Background Noise All But Disappears 67
Types of Assistive Listening Devices 69
    1. Personal Amplifiers 70
    2. FM Systems 71
    3. Infrared Systems 71
    4. Induction Loop Systems 72
    5. Bluetooth Systems 73
Amplified Telephones 73
Connecting Your Hearing Aids to Assistive Devices 74
    T-coils 74
    Direct Audio Input (DAI) 74
    FM Receivers 75
    Bluetooth 75
The Last Word 75

Good Books on Hearing Loss 77

About the Author

Neil G. Bauman, Ph.D., (Dr. Neil), is the executive director of the Center for Hearing Loss Help. He is a hearing loss coping skills specialist, researcher, author and speaker on issues pertaining to hearing loss. No stranger to hearing loss himself, he has lived with a life-long severe hereditary hearing loss.

Dr. Neil did not let his hearing loss stop him from achieving what he wanted to do. He earned several degrees in fields ranging from forestry to ancient astronomy (Ph. D.) and theology (Th. D.), in addition to his extensive studies in fields related to hearing loss.

His mission is helping hard of hearing people understand and successfully cope with their hearing losses and other ear conditions. To this end, he provides education, support and counsel to hard of hearing people through personal contact, as well as through his books, articles, presentations and seminars.

Dr. Neil is the author of eleven books and more than six hundred articles on hearing-loss related topics. (See the back of this book for a list of his books.) In addition, he is a dynamic speaker. His presentations are in demand throughout the USA and Canada.

You can reach him at:

Neil Bauman, Ph.D.
Center for Hearing Loss Help
49 Piston Court
Stewartstown, PA 17363
Phone: (717) 993-8555
FAX: (717) 993-6661
Email: neil@hearinglosshelp.com
Web site: http://www.hearinglosshelp.com

Introduction

Hearing Loss Upsets the Apple Cart!

When hearing loss strikes us, it upsets our "Apple Carts." This is what happened to Bena. (Incidentally, the stories I'll be telling you throughout this session are true—they all happened to people I know.)

Bena suddenly she sat bolt upright, her eyes riveted to the clock. That couldn't be right. Why hadn't the alarm wakened her? She would be late for work! She jumped out of bed and dashed to the bathroom. The house was eerily silent. The water splashed silently into the basin. Something was dreadfully wrong. Then it struck her. She couldn't hear a sound. She had gone to bed with normal hearing, and sometime during the night she had lost all her hearing as she slept. Now she was deaf!

Not everyone has such a dramatic introduction to hearing loss as Bena had. To be sure, hearing loss comes from many causes and strikes at any age. For example, Doreen suddenly lost her hearing one day while teaching in school because a blood clot lodged in her neck. In contrast, Delmar, another teacher, had his hearing loss sneak up on him so gradually over several years that he didn't even realize that he was losing his hearing until his superintendent pointed out that he wasn't hearing his students' questions anymore.

Bonnie lost her hearing from taking an antibiotic to fight a life-threatening infection. Vera lost her hearing as a girl from the effects of meningitis. Vern slowly lost his hearing from working in a noisy machine shop. Becky lost her hearing at birth when the umbilical cord wrapped around her neck and temporarily cut off the oxygen supply to her brain. Marguerite lost her hearing as she grew older. Andy lost his on the farm working with noisy tractors. Sam lost his from repeated, severe middle ear infections as he was growing up. Lynn lost hers before birth when her mother contracted rubella (German measles). Shawn lost his from a brain tumor operation. I was born with an inherited hearing loss.

However, for the vast majority of you, hearing loss sneaks up on you so gradually over several months or years, or even decades, that you aren't even aware you are losing your hearing.

The truth is, hard of hearing people are often the **last** ones to realize they have hearing losses. They are too busy blaming their communication difficulties on others. This was the case with "Harry" and his wife (see box below).

Spaghetti and Meatballs

"Harry" was concerned that his wife, "Betty," was losing her hearing although Betty heatedly denied it. Exasperated, Harry went to an ear specialist. "Doctor," he said, "What can I do to prove to my wife that she needs to get her hearing attended to?"

The specialist suggested, "Stand some distance behind her and ask her a question. If she doesn't answer, keep moving closer and repeating the question until she answers. Then you will know just how bad her hearing is."

Later, at home, "Harry" saw "Betty" making supper at the kitchen counter. From the living room he called, "Honey, what are we having for dinner?" As he expected, there was no reply.

So he moved closer—into the dining room—and called again, "Honey, what's for dinner?" Still no reply.

He moved still closer, stood in the kitchen doorway, and asked for the third time, "Honey, what's for dinner?" He was shocked when again there was no reply. He hadn't thought her hearing was **that** bad.

Finally, moving up behind her, he asked yet again, "Honey, what's for dinner?"

Turning to face him she answered, "Spaghetti and meat balls—I said—for the fourth time!"

No matter how you lose your hearing, or how fast or slow it occurs—the end result is the same—**you** join the ranks of hard of hearing people. The big question is, "**What do I do now?**"

Six Keys to Successfully Living with Your Hearing Loss

This is where this book is going to help you. There are six basic keys to successfully learning to live with your hearing loss. They are:

1. Psychologically adjust to your hearing loss, including grieving for your hearing loss. This includes both you and your family, as hearing loss affects communication with everyone around you.

2. Learn to cope with your hearing loss the right way. This includes understanding why you act the way you do.

3. Learn, and put into practice, good coping skills and strategies. There are many, many of these. The nice thing about most of these is that not only do they work, but they are also **free**! You can use them any time and any place.

4. Learn to speechread. (Lip reading was the older term.)

5. Get and wear properly fitted hearing aids if they will help you. If your hearing is too poor for hearing aids, consider getting cochlear implants.

6. Supplement your hearing aids with Assistive Technology in those areas where hearing aids aren't very effective.

Unfortunately, when hearing loss strikes, most people think that all they need to do is get hearing aids and their hearing will be all "hunky dory" again, but this is just not true. Hearing aids are only **part** of the solution. Like their name implies, hearing aids are **aids** to hearing, not cures for hearing loss. Thus, you need to use all six of these keys, not just one, if you want to successfully live with your hearing loss.

Chapter 1

The Critical Missing Element to Successfully Living with Your Hearing Loss—Grieving for Your Hearing Loss

When we lose some, much, or all of our hearing, especially if it is reasonably sudden, we are thrown into emotional turmoil whether we admit it or not—and we men often won't admit it.

We cope with our losses one way or another. Some of us do the right things, but unfortunately, many of us, at least initially, cope the wrong way—like Robin did. Here is her story.

Robin was a normal-hearing, 21-year-old young woman when she went to a sleep-over at a friend's house. Due to a tragic set of circumstances, she awoke the next morning totally deaf. She relates,

> "I walked out of my friend's house to get a ride home—they lived on a highway—and I saw a tractor-trailer go whizzing by, the trees, leaves and grass bending and swaying as the truck raced past me, but there was no sound. The lack of sound just did not compute to my brain. I was numb."

The tragedy of losing her hearing overnight turned Robin into a zombie as she struggled to deal with her loss.

What did she do? She explained,

> "I shut myself up in my bedroom for 20 months!"

Why? She continued,

"I didn't know how to deal with this hearing loss. I didn't know anyone else who was hard of hearing. Furthermore, I refused to consider hearing aids."

No matter how you lose your hearing, once you become aware of your hearing loss, what you do next largely determines whether you will live a happy, fulfilled life as a hard of hearing person, or whether you have just set yourself up for all sorts of physical, emotional and psychological problems in the future like Robin did.

You don't have to be like Robin. You **can** successfully live with your hearing loss.

So what are you supposed to do? You need to work though this first key step (and one so many people miss) and work though the grieving process in regards to your hearing loss.

What Is Grief?

Grief is intense emotional suffering caused by a significant loss in our lives. We valued our hearing. Therefore, we quite naturally grieve when we lose it. Our grief shows that we recognize we have a hearing loss and that we are powerless to restore it.

This is much the same as if our spouse died. There is nothing we can do to get him or her back. We are powerless to do anything about it—so we grieve.

Grieving actually is a **process** we work through, not a state of being. Did you get that? It is important that you understand that grieving is a **process**, and you work though a process. It has a beginning and an end. It does not last forever.

Furthermore, the grieving process is a natural, necessary, healthy condition that includes a number of emotional safety valves to release the pressure so we don't "blow up" or "melt down". You **need** to grieve. It is **not** optional if you want to successfully live with your hearing loss.

No one denies that grieving is painful, and we don't like to be in pain, do we? Thus, it is natural that we try to shrink away from the grieving process. This is wrong. We need to embrace the grieving process, work though it and get on with our lives.

When we squarely face our hearing loss, the waves of emotions and feelings we call grief flow over us. Like the waves of the sea, this grieving process can't be rushed, and it can't be turned back. These waves of grief will continue to wash over us for some time, but slowly they will get less and less, and finally they will subside. Fear, sadness, crying and thinking about our loss are all normal expressions of grief.

The Stages of Grief

When we lose some of our hearing as adults, many of us experience the same emotional shock and grief we would if we learned that we had a terminal illness. In her book *On Death and Dying* (published in 1969), psychiatrist Elisabeth Kubler-Ross explained the five stages of grief that terminally-ill people go through—denial, anger, bargaining, depression and acceptance.

People with hearing loss advance through these same five stages of grief as they say goodbye to the hearing they once enjoyed and prepare themselves for their new lives as hard of hearing people. Saying "Good bye" to the old life, and saying "Hello" to the new life, is the essence of the grieving process.

Each of us progress through these stages at our own pace. For some, it may take a few days. For others, it may take several years.

Realize that this is not a cut and dried process. We are not necessarily only in one stage of the grieving process at any given time. For example, we can still be in denial in one aspect of our hearing loss, while perfectly accepting of it in another. Likewise, we can be angry over one area affected by our lack of hearing, and be depressed in another area at the same time.

Furthermore, we may skip one or more of these stages of grief, or go through them in a different order. Also, we may regress and go through certain stages over and over again. This is especially true if we have progressive hearing losses. For example, "Jerri" explained,

> "I'm still in the grieving process. The problem is that anytime I get better and start to lead a normal life, my hearing gets worse, and down I go again! It's been a hectic emotional roller coaster."

Here are the five stages of grief and how they may affect us as we progress through them.

Denial

The news shocks us. Maybe we went to the doctor, or took a child to the doctor, and his diagnosis is severe hearing loss. We express disbelief. "It can't be!" "They're wrong!" "It's not me they are talking about!" "Someone made a mistake!" "I don't have a hearing loss!"

Denial is our first, and perfectly natural, reaction when faced with the shocking news we have a hearing loss. Often, it is too painful for us to accept that we will never again hear better than we do now.

Consequently, we may be shocked numb just like Robin. The shock temporarily anesthetizes us—gives us a brief escape from reality. We may show little emotion at this point. This shock stage may last anywhere from a few minutes to a few hours to a few days.

By temporarily blocking out our loss, we give ourselves time to adjust more gradually to our new reality. We need denial temporarily, but we must not linger on it. If we linger it becomes a lie, not just an emotional shock-absorber.

Eventually, it becomes obvious to us that we really do have a hearing loss and that we cannot deny it any longer. Our next reaction is to deny its permanence. Now, instead of saying, "I don't have a hearing loss," we tell ourselves and others that our hearing losses are just temporary. Soon a doctor will discover a miraculous cure like hair cell regeneration or a magic pill, and we will be able to hear normally again.

Some people linger in this denial stage for years. It is important to understand that you will not do much, if anything, about your hearing loss until you are emotionally/psychologically ready. This will **never** happen as long as you are in the denial stage. Why should you do anything about a hearing loss you deny you even have?

Anger

Once we admit we have a hearing loss, we often experience rage or anger, and even envy and resentment, especially if we experienced a relatively sudden hearing loss. We ask, "Why me?" "It just isn't fair!" "God, what did I do that you are punishing me with a hearing loss?"

In our anger, we may become stubborn, rebellious, abusive and destructive. This doesn't make it right. I'm just explaining the emotions we are going through. We may deny these negative traits in ourselves, and instead, project them upon others.

We often feel robbed, resentful and angry with ourselves or anything that caused our hearing loss. In this state of mind, we may lash out at everyone and everything. If you are a family member, don't take it personally. This is a process your loved one must work through.

Bargaining

After we quit denying our hearing loss, and after our anger has subsided, we may try to bargain with ourselves, with our doctors or with God for the return of our hearing. We are more inclined to bargain if we do not perceive our hearing loss as being permanent. Bargaining seldom works because what have we to bargain with?

Depression

Denial has not worked. We are still "deaf". Anger has not worked. We are still hard of hearing. Bargaining has not worked. We still can't hear. Thus we conclude that nothing works. We **finally** realize that our hearing loss is real and is not going away. This depresses us. This stage represents a kind of giving up the fight. We acknowledge it is futile to continue fighting.

We may feel varying degrees of sadness, loneliness and despair. We may feel that life is not worth living any more. We may wish we were dead. We may say to ourselves, "I couldn't care less." Thus, our usual activities lose their importance. Our hearing losses make us feel insecure and isolated. Consequently, we withdraw from many social situations. Furthermore, during this stage, we do not feel like doing anything to help ourselves hear better. We have reached rock bottom. At this point, there doesn't seem to be any hope at all.

If you want to break the grieving process into two parts, the first part—up to now—is all downhill—heading for rock bottom. The good news is that once we reach rock bottom there is only one way to go—up.

A surprising thing now happens. We begin to see the light at the end of the tunnel, so to speak. Think of it this way. The grieving process is like entering a long, dark tunnel. We can't see anything in front of us. We think we are stuck in the blackness forever.

What we don't know is that this tunnel is curved, and after we have gotten to the half-way point, by just taking a few more steps, we can see around the bend—and there it is—the light at the end of the tunnel! From here on, gradually our depression and sadness lessens and the darkness begins to lift as more and more light floods our tunnel.

It is at this point that we begin taking steps—perhaps tiny ones at first—toward becoming involved in life again. It may take from several months to two years or more to finally come to this stage. We may begin to fantasize, and in our dream world, put ourselves into many different situations to see how we can fit in. This is a positive step. As we meet each new little challenge, we learn to handle our hearing losses, and our depression begins to lift.

Unfortunately, some people stay in the depression stage for a number of years. It's as if they stop and give up just before they reach the middle of the tunnel—afraid to go on. That is why it is so important for each of us to have a person who has been down this road before, to guide us and to support us. We need someone that can tell us about that wonderful curve in the middle of the tunnel; someone that can reassure us that what we are experiencing is normal; someone that can let us know we are making progress in the grieving process, so we are encouraged to continue to press on to success.

Acceptance

The final stage is acceptance. In this stage, we now concentrate more on the future than sorrowing over the past. We are in the final few feet of the tunnel heading towards the light. It is in this stage that we begin to look for ways to successfully cope with our hearing losses. Unfortunately, no matter how well we cope with our hearing losses, there will always be some activities we just won't be able to handle as before. Thus, our lifestyles will change, but note this well; **they need not be any less worthwhile or rewarding—just different**.

We have reached the acceptance stage when we freely admit, "There is something wrong with my hearing, not with me. I am okay. Only my hearing is impaired, not my intelligence. I may not feel good about being hard of hearing, but I do feel good about myself. You begin thinking of ways to cope with your hearing loss. You are open to help and advice now. As you put coping strategies into place, you say to yourself, "I don't want to miss out on things any more. Even if I can't hear very well, I still want to enjoy life to its fullest. I **am** going to live again!" At this point, you have successfully made it through the whole grieving process. **That** is success.

The Rest of the Family Needs to Grieve Too

So far, we have just looked at how hearing loss affects us. Unfortunately, when hearing loss hits one family member, it affects everyone in the family, not just the person with the hearing loss. Typically, the other family members miss the free and easy (and intimate) conversations they used to have. This saddens and sometimes angers them. Thus, just as for any other kind of loss, they too have to grieve this loss.

Be aware that when parents discover that their child has a hearing loss, it can hit them hard—as it did Tom and his wife—almost as if their child had died. In fact, this is exactly what they may feel—that the "normal" hearing child they gave birth to has "died," leaving in its place a "deaf" child. Thus, their grief is very real, and they need time to grieve.

Hearing loss in the family can hit children hard too. When sudden severe hearing loss hit the mother in one family, her young daughter had a tough time dealing with it. Her daughter remembers the day her mother was taken to the hospital. She sadly lamented,

> "Mommy came back a different mommy. I lost my old mommy. This mommy can't hear. I want my old Mommy back!"

Because she did not have proper support, this little girl regressed. She became a bed wetter and began to have temper tantrums. Thus, when hearing loss hits a family, never forget the needs of the children. They need an external support network to help them through their grief. The reason children need external support is because when their parents are mired in their own grief, they cannot effectively help their children.

If hearing loss hits a spouse, and both do not grieve this loss of communication, it often causes a great strain in the marriage. In fact, unless they work through the grieving process, many marriages do not survive.

Part of the problem is that since both marriage partners need to grieve, they are not available to support each other. The person with the hearing loss is busy grieving and needs support. However, the person they turn too in their grief—their husband or wife—is also grieving, and thus cannot effectively help them. That is why it is **vital** that both the hard of hearing spouse and the hearing spouse **each** have their own support networks to help them successfully navigate the grieving process.

This is what "Sally" and "Bill" did. Sally explained,

> "Bill and I couldn't support each other in the beginning. We were weighed down by our own sadness and grief. It was like we were sinking because the two of us together were too heavy for our marriage boat. At this point, I turned to my friends, and Bill turned to his. As a result, we stayed together, but we really did have to go outside of our marriage for support."

When Is the Right Time to Get Hearing Aids?
Where Do Hearing Aids Fit into the Grieving Process?

If your doctor or audiologist has just diagnosed you with a significant hearing loss, **don't** rush out and buy yourself new hearing aids. Pay attention here, because there is a right and a wrong time to get hearing aids. Here's a typical scenario.

You come home with the shocking diagnosis—you have a hearing loss. The first reaction of your hearing family members is to pressure you into getting hearing aids.

Family members, resist this temptation. Yes, your spouse needs hearing aids. However, this is **not** the right time for him/her to get hearing aids. The truth is, millions of dollars of hearing aids lay abandoned in dresser drawers—unwanted and unused—because family members pressured hard of hearing people into getting hearing aids **before** they were ready. Let me explain why in relation to the grieving process.

Denial: Your wife drags you in to have your hearing tested and to hopefully be fitted with hearing aids, because she is convinced you are losing your hearing. However, as far as you are concerned, it is a total waste of time because you **know** you still hear perfectly fine, so you don't need hearing aids.

Family member, put yourself in the hard of hearing person's shoes. Would you wear hearing aids if you "knew" your hearing was still okay? Of course not! Thus, if you "force" your spouse to get hearing aids, he will often just give his new hearing aids a cursory trial, take them home, toss them in a dresser drawer, and forget all about them. And there goes $5,000.00 down the drain!

Anger: In this stage you are **mad**! When you are mad, you are not thinking rationally. You notice that people aren't speaking up. It's them, not you. You don't need hearing aids! People just need to learn to speak up properly! You think, "Why spend money on hearing aids when your communications problems are not even your fault?"

Bargaining: You have now accepted the fact that you really do have a hearing loss, but you "know" this loss is going to be temporary. You are going to work a deal with the doctors, or maybe even with God Himself, to get your hearing back. Since your hearing loss is going to be temporary, why should you waste good money buying hearing aids you're hardly ever going to use?

Depression: When none of the above works, you become depressed. Since you are depressed, you feel that life is no longer worth living, so what difference does it make whether you hear better or not? Thus, you still won't bother with hearing aids.

Acceptance: Finally, however, you begin to realize that you **want** to live life to its fullest and to do that you need to hear better. It is at this point that you are ready to do whatever it takes in order to hear better. Now is the time for you to hurry to your audiologist for your new hearing aids, because now you are finally ready and willing to give them a fair trial.

Book to Help You in the Grieving Process

The grieving process is a most important step in becoming well-adjusted to your hearing loss. So important, in fact, that you need more than the brief overview I've given you here, especially if you don't have anyone to guide you through the grieving process.

I highly recommend the short, easy-to-read book ***Grieving for Your Hearing Loss—The Rocky Road from Denial to Acceptance***. (See page 80.) This little book has helped many effectively deal with their hearing losses.

Here are some real-life examples.

"Nora" wrote, "A few months ago I ordered Dr. Neil's book on grieving. I really cried when I read it—good tears! I felt as if someone finally understood what I was going through. He is so right! We do need to work through the various stages of grieving."

"Cindy" said, "I just read Neil's book on grieving and found it to be extremely helpful since I seem to be losing my hearing by drips and drabs. I keep going through this grieving process over and over and over—every time my hearing decreases."

"Wendy" declared, "I wholeheartedly recommend this book. It helped my husband and me. One of the things I realized was that my husband and I were so stuck in our sadness and grief that we couldn't see the forest for the trees."

"Daisy" exclaimed, "Neil, I just finished reading your book ***Grieving for Your Hearing Loss***. It was great! At first I didn't think this book was for me, but as I read on, I saw a description of myself! I have recently entered the acceptance stage. Things have been changing for the better ever since."

If you are going through the grieving process, things can change for the better for you too! You can go on-line and purchase a copy of this grieving book for yourself at **http://www.hearinglosshelp.com/products/books.htm**. Put yourself on the road to hope and recovery now.

Chapter 2

Coping with Hearing Loss the Right Way!— Why We Act the Way We Do

In this chapter we are going to delve into the psychology of hearing loss and learn how we can learn to make good communication choices day after day.

Coping Outcomes

Whenever we communicate, we typically employ various hearing loss coping strategies that we hope will help us communicate better.

These coping strategies can have one of three outcomes. Either they will:

1. Improve the situation (good coping strategies) or

2. Leave the situation unchanged (ineffective coping strategies) or

3. Make the situation worse (bad coping strategies).

You would think that because we can't hear well, we would always take steps to make the communication situation better, wouldn't you?

Surprise! It doesn't work out that way in real life. The shocking truth is that for the first few years after our hearing losses, and perhaps for a long time after that, we **habitually** react to communication problems in ways that tend to **make the situation worse** rather than better. Can you believe it?

The question is, "Why do we so often make the communication situation worse, rather than better?" The answer is that our human nature subconsciously gets in the way and subverts our sincere efforts to cope properly. The good news is that once we are aware of what is going on, we can actively choose to make good hearing loss coping strategy decisions.

We Often Use Emotion-Focused Rather Than Problem-Focused Coping Strategies

There are two basic ways we can solve our communication problems. Either we are **emotion-focused,** or we are **problem-focused**. Which one we choose makes all the difference in the outcome.

The main reason that emotion-focused coping strategies don't work is because the goal of **emotion-focused** coping strategies is **not to hear better**, but to **feel better**. In contrast, the goal of **problem-focused** coping strategies is to **solve the communication problem** and not worry about our feelings in the process.

Unfortunately, because we are human, we tend to focus more on things that make us **feel better** rather than strategies that will help us hear better—**especially** if solving the problem is going to make us temporarily feel worse.

Example 1: Not Hearing at a Meeting

Let me give you an example. You are at a meeting—one that you thought was going to be a lecture, but it turns out that the speaker (namely me) is picking on people in the audience and asking them questions. Let's say you can't hear me too well, and as the minutes tick by you grow more and more anxious and apprehensive that I'm going to ask you a question. You are worried that either you won't know the answer (and thus will look stupid in public), or you are worried that you won't hear and understand the question because of your poor hearing (and again look stupid in public), not to mention causing you acute embarrassment in the process.

The Wrong Way

As the meeting progresses, your anxiety level rises higher and higher. You refuse to make eye contact with me, hoping against hope that I won't pick on you. (And if you're not making eye contact with me, then you are leaving out one of the five basic key hearing loss coping strategies—speechreading.) All you want to do is sink through the floor. Since you can't do that, you do the one thing that you can do to help you feel better. You make some excuse to the person beside you, get up and hurry from the meeting, probably never to return.

Was this action an emotion-focused or problem-focused strategy? (You didn't leave the room in order to hear better!)

Right—it was emotion-focused. You did this in order to **feel better**. By quickly leaving, you gained relief from the terrible anxiety you were feeling.

This solved your emotional problem for the moment—gaining relief from your increasing anxiety—but it did nothing to solve the basic communication problem—namely not being able to adequately hear the speaker. Nor did it help you to feel good about yourself. Instead of advocating for yourself, you just ran away.

The result is that you probably now feel even worse because you still don't know what was being said, which, after all, was your whole purpose in coming to this meeting in the first place. Add to that, you know you chickened out, thus your feelings of self-worth and self-esteem dropped another notch.

All in all, it was a losing strategy. You lost the whole content of the meeting and you lost some more self-esteem. It's just not worth it for saving a few moments of anxiety when there is a better way to do it.

The Right Way

Now let's look at how you could have better solved this communication problem if you had been problem-focused instead of emotion-focused.

There are two aspects—what you can do for yourself and what you need others to do to help you.

First, you need to do what you can do for yourself in order to make the communication situation better. For example, if you are not sitting in the front row, you could get up and move to where you can hear better. Are you wearing your hearing aids or using the proper assistive listening devices? Don't expect other people to help you hear better until you are doing everything you can do to help yourself.

Second, let's look at what you could have done to enlist the help of others. For example, you could have interrupted me (the speaker) and explained that you have trouble hearing, thus you need me to talk a little louder, or a little slower, or to repeat the questions and comments from the audience—or whatever your need is at the moment. You might ask me to stand in one place facing you instead of pacing the platform.

The real question is, "Why don't you do these things?" The answer is plain and simple—you're too embarrassed! Doing any of these things would call attention both to yourself and to your hearing loss, and would make you **feel worse**, not better, right at that moment. You see, a lot of people think it is somehow shameful to admit to having a hearing loss. They feel there is a stigma attached to having a hearing loss. So you sit quietly in your seat. You say nothing. You do nothing!

In contrast, let's say you do one or more of these coping strategies. Now you are effectively addressing, and resolving, the basic communication problem. This is **problem-focused** coping behavior.

Guess what happens when you do this? First, after the initial embarrassment passes, you will feel better because now you can hear what you wanted to hear. Second, your anxiety level drops. Also, you have let everyone know that you are not stupid, but just have a hearing loss, so people are going to have a better opinion of you. Finally, your feelings of self-worth and self-esteem jump up a notch.

You see, not only do problem-focused coping strategies solve the communication problem, as a side benefit, problem-focused coping efforts help to **increase our self-esteem** because we have done something that solved a problem in a positive way.

However, sometimes it's just not possible to resolve the underlying communication problem. (Remember, communication is a two-way street. Both the speaker **and** the listener have to be involved.) Maybe the speaker refuses to speak up, or maybe he has an accent we just can't understand, and there are no handouts or real-time captioning available. In these cases, we need to focus on finding ways to reduce our emotional distress.

At this point, we may realize that it is hopeless to stay and hear nothing, so we get up and walk out. This is a **right** use of emotion-focused coping behavior. Using it this way, we work to reduce any **needless** emotional wear and tear on ourselves. Notice the key—needless emotional wear and tear. We should only use this as a last resort!

Another coping strategy at this point when you can't hear the speaker is to come prepared and bring a book to read, or your knitting like my wife does, until you come to a part of the meeting that you can hear.

When we use emotion-focused strategies we **never** learn proper problem-solving coping strategies. We need to do our best to use the problem-focused coping strategies first, and then, if they don't work, switch to the emotion-focused coping strategies.

Let me tell you a story about a problem-focused effective communication strategy I used. I used to be in Toastmasters—in fact I am a Distinguished Toastmaster. One day a man from India, Hitesh by name, joined our club. The problem was he spoke with a heavy Indian accent, and I couldn't understand him. That wasn't the worst of it. Since I was one of the top speakers in my club, and have a number of trophies to show for it, he wanted me to coach him to become a better speaker! Between my poor ears and his strong accent that was an impossible situation—so I said, "Sure! I'll help you," because I quickly figured out a way that I could help him in spite of not being able to understand his speech.

I told him, "E-mail me your speeches, and I'll critique them via e-mail." This worked, and his speeches improved although when he presented them at Toastmasters, I still couldn't understand what he was saying! So always look for ways you can solve communication problems. As they say, "where there's a will, there's a way!"

The **major problem** associated with using **emotion-focused** coping strategies is that we **face the same problems time after time** with the same dismal results. We never learn effective problem-focused coping strategies.

This causes us to have a pessimistic attitude. We keep on trying, but by inadvertently doing the same wrong things over and over again, we perpetuate, or worsen, the communication problems.

In these circumstances, it is easy to blame other people for our problems by labeling them insensitive, uncaring, or stubborn. It is so easy for us to then give up trying. When this happens we will **never** successfully live with our hearing losses.

How much better to continually practice problem-focused coping strategies. Some people will learn. The truth is, a lot of people just plain forget about your hearing needs, so you have to keep on reminding them until they "get it".

Not everyone is uncaring and insensitive. For example, at one of my Toastmaster club meetings, the speaker was going to give a presentation using an overhead projector and turned off the lights. Quickly another Toastmaster spoke up, "Turn the lights back on. Neil needs the light in order to speechread

27

you." I just about fell off my chair I was so surprised! Not only did I get to hear without having to advocate for myself yet again, but my feelings of self-esteem went up a notch. Someone thought enough of me and my hearing loss to make sure I could hear! Another win-win situation.

Example 2: Bluffing

Because we fail to use proper coping strategies to overcome our hearing losses, we may resort to using an all-time favorite, yet totally wrong, coping strategy—one that is used by every hard of hearing person the world over at one time or another. That strategy is **bluffing**. Bluffing is simply pretending to hear and understand when you don't have a clue what people are saying.

Just because bluffing is common and we all do it, it doesn't mean it is okay. It is still wrong!

Typically bluffing includes such things as nodding and smiling, and saying "uh huh."

Mrs. G_____ had her bluffing down pat. Whenever the speaker's mouth went up in a smile she said, "Yes, yes!" Whenever the speaker's mouth went down in a frown, she said, "What a pity." When you are bluffing, there is no real communication taking place, although you can fool many people, at least part of the time.

When you bluff and respond inappropriately, this just reinforces in the hearing person's mind their view that you (and all hard of hearing people) are indeed stupid and incompetent.

Here is an example of what I mean. One hard of hearing young woman had a mortifying experience on a noisy bus. A woman sitting opposite had started talking to her, and she couldn't understand a word. She responded in her usual manner by bluffing: "Oh yes, certainly, uh huh, that's true", etc. Finally the woman stood up, shouted at her angrily, spat her gum on the floor and left. She hadn't been talking at all. She'd been chewing gum!

Imagine the embarrassment this lady felt after that emotion-focused coping strategy blew up in her face. That alone is one good reason to determine **never** to bluff; besides bluffing is lying, and lying is always wrong!

Bluffing is **always** an **emotion-focused** strategy, never a problem-focused one. That alone tells you it is not going to be effective in solving communication problems.

How much better to be up-front about your hearing loss and your unique communication needs. Keep your sense of humor when you do it. Sharon, who is hard of hearing, is problem-focused. She explained, "When I met a whole room-full of strangers at a new symphonic band I joined, I asked for a couple of minutes, and told everyone, 'I am hard of hearing. If I tell you how sorry I am to hear about your promotion, or congratulate you on a death in the family, please don't take it personally!'" Everyone roared. All the subsequent bloopers she made were forgiven in advance—and she made many!

Let's look at an example of bluffing, and then look at the correct way to handle this situation. Here's the scenario.

The Wrong Way

I am walking down the sidewalk and a person is approaching me. As he gets closer, he says something that sounds sort of like "wa I ih ih." I don't have a clue what he just said, so I do what the typical hard of hearing person does, I bluff. I just nod and smile at him, hoping that that will satisfy him, but it doesn't.

He again says, "wa I ih ih". By now my embarrassment and anxiety levels are beginning to skyrocket. I nod and smile again—hoping against hope it will work this time.

But he becomes even more insistent. I know he wants something, and I don't have a clue what he wants. My anxiety level is now well into the stratosphere. I **need** to get away fast to curb my enormous anxiety. (Notice how emotion-focused I am at this point. I'm worrying about how I am feeling, not about solving the communication problem.)

Desperately I try to come up with some solution to this situation. I pointedly look at my watch, mutter that I am late for a meeting or something, and hurry away.

What is the result of this emotion-focused coping strategy?

1. I have deprived myself of an opportunity to practice effective problem-focused communication behavior—identifying the problem and suggesting ways of overcoming it.

2. The longer I bluff, the more anxious and embarrassed I become.

3. I risk the other person becoming angry at me when he finds out I haven't understood anything he said and haven't told him.

4. I make myself look stupid. I have just reinforced this stranger's opinion that hard of hearing people are both stupid and lacking in the social graces.

5. I am mad at myself for being so wimpy, and my self-esteem plummets. I feel worse about myself in the long term—not better.

Overall, it was a lose-lose situation.

What have I learned? Absolutely nothing about effective communication. All I've learned is that I get anxious around people so I may try to avoid them in the future. No wonder so many hard of hearing people take anti-anxiety medications! Furthermore, I'm feeling worse about myself, so now I need to take anti-depressant drugs also.

The truth is, these drugs aren't necessary. All we need to do is learn proper problem-solving hearing loss coping strategies and then use them. The more you use them, the easier it gets.

The Right Way

Now let's play this same scenario again, but this time I am going to use problem-focused coping strategies. Notice how different the outcome is.

I am walking down the sidewalk again, and a person is approaching me. As he gets closer, he says something that sounds sort of like "wa I ih ih." I don't have a clue what he just said, but I think I may get it the next time, so I say, "What was that again?" and again he goes "wa I ih ih". I still didn't catch any more of it.

Now it is the height of stupidity to do the same thing over and over again and expect a different result each time. I quickly realize that I need to use a different coping strategy in order to solve this communication problem because simple repetition isn't working.

So I say to him, "I know you are asking me something, but I have a hearing loss and didn't understand what you said. I need you to stop, look at me and speak a bit louder and more slowly." While I am saying this, I am walking right up to him, and now am standing nose to nose so to speak.

Notice what I have done. This is critically important. I have told him I am hard of hearing. Telling a person you have a hearing loss is good. It lets them know there is a communication problem, but it is not enough. In the same breath, I then told him what I needed him to do at that point so we could have a successful communication. Too often we don't tell the other person what we need them to do—and the typical hearing person doesn't know what they need to do. The result is they too become anxious. Now you have two emotion-focused people. The result is that the chances of having a successful communication is slim.

Also notice that I did what I could. I got close to him so I could both hear and speechread.

This time when he speaks, I catch the word "time" and say, "Oh, are you asking me what time it is?" At his nod, I look at my watch and tell him.

You see what I heard was "wa I ih ih?" but with my poor hearing I missed the high-frequency consonants. What he really had said was, "What time is it?"

Let's look at the results of using the problem-focused approach.

1. The other person's is now happy—he knows the answer to his question.

2. He has learned that hard of hearing people aren't stupid. They just have problems hearing.

3. He has also learned that in order to effectively communicate with hard of hearing people he needs to do certain things such as get close, face them, speak up and speak slowly and clearly.

From my perspective as a hard of hearing person, what have I learned?

1. When using problem-focused coping strategies, my anxiety level stays more or less on an even keel.

2. Problem-focused coping strategies actually work.

3. I feel good about myself—I have helped a fellow human being. My feelings of self-worth and self-esteem rise. (I don't need any anti-anxiety drugs or anti-depressants!)

Overall, it is a win-win situation. This is how important it is to practice problem-focused coping strategies rather than emotion-focused coping strategies.

Always Think, "Are the Benefits Worth the Costs?"

We have just seen why people habitually resort to behaviors that not only fail to resolve communication problems, but also frequently serve to make the situation worse. The reason is, they are emotion-focused rather than problem-focused.

Now we need to ask, "What motivates such behavior?" There has to be some payoff for these reactions or people wouldn't persist in resorting to them.

We have to ask ourselves, "**Are the short-term costs worth the long-term benefits?**" When we do this we are using problem-focused coping strategies.

Unfortunately, we so often **want short term benefits**, and we never give a thought to the long term costs. This is what happens when we let emotion-focused behavior take over.

Let me use, as an example, another one of our favorite ploys—dominating the conversation.

Let's break it down and first look at the short term benefits. When we dominate the conversation we:

>... don't have to wonder what the topic is, nor what people are saying—since we are doing all of it.

>... don't have to strain to hear since we are the only one doing the talking.

>... don't feel anxious. Our anxiety level is low.

Those look like a bunch of good benefits—and they all make us feel better in the short term.

Now let's look at the long-term costs. When we dominate the conversation, we lose our friends. No one wants to talk with us, because they know they won't be able to get a word in edgewise. Thus we end up shunned and lonely. Our feelings of self-esteem and self-worth drop and we end up depressed.

When we look at it carefully, it is **not** worth trading the short-term benefits for these long-term costs.

Now let's look at how we could use problem-focused coping strategies so that the long-term benefits far outweigh the short term costs.

Instead of filibustering and dominating the conversation, we could speak up and say, "Hey, guys, I have a hearing loss and am having a lot of trouble following this conversation. Would you mind talking one at a time? And would you mind repeating a few things I missed? Or would you mind speaking into my microphone?"

Now what you have traded off is a short-term cost of being slightly embarrassed for interrupting your friends, but you have gained the long-term benefit of still having the same friends 10 or 20 years later. You are not going to be lonely. And because you have effectively advocated for your hearing needs, you feel good about yourself. Thus your feelings of self-worth and self-esteem rise.

I think you can now see that when we use **emotion-focused** coping strategies, we typically only look at the **short-term benefits** and **not** the **long-term costs**, or without thinking, we **imagine** the short term benefits far outweigh the long-term costs.

You see, our human minds are wired to be more concerned about our current comfort levels (short-term benefits) than with the long-term costs. Thus, when we make decisions, we often act as if the future doesn't exist—or at least doesn't count for very much.

However, when we sit down and carefully evaluate the situation, we soon realize that emotion-focused coping strategies actually have questionable short-term benefits, but **enormous** long-term costs. In other words, **emotion-focused** coping strategies are just **not** worth it when you really think about it.

In conclusion, if there's only one thing you remember from this chapter, **always beware of emotion-focused coping efforts that produce short-term benefits (require less effort, or reduce personal discomfort) but have long-term costs (reduced self-esteem and damaged relationships)**.

Instead, we need to consciously choose **problem-focused** coping strategies. When we do this, the ultimate results will be reduced anxiety, increased self-esteem and easier communication—and **that's** something worth striving for!

Chapter 3

Seven Effective and Free Hearing Loss Coping Strategies

I was born with a severe hearing loss. As a result, I had to learn how to cope with my hearing loss from day one. What I'll be explaining in this chapter isn't some ivory tower theory, but the practical, down-to-earth, everyday things I use to successfully cope with my hearing loss. If you or someone you know has a hearing loss, the strategies you learn in this chapter will help you, and them, better cope with hearing loss.

1. The Single Most Effective Hearing Loss Coping Strategy—Get Close!

If you only had one coping strategy you could employ, and it mustn't cost a cent, what would this single most effective hearing loss coping strategy be?

Yes, that strategy is: **get close—get as close as you can to the speaker**.

You see, when you have a hearing loss, distance is your enemy! Never forget it. In order to hear and understand speech, we need to be close. Few people realize just how critical distance is in our ability to understand speech. An ideal distance for conversing with a hard of hearing person is how much?—just 3 to 6 feet! That's it. At that distance, our hearing aids will pick up your voice the best, we will be able to speechread you clearly and background noise won't bother us much.

There are **four very good reasons** to get close.

1.1 Sounds Drop Off with Increasing Distance

Sounds get softer the further you are from the speaker. You all know this, but do you realize just how dramatic this drop off is? If I am talking and you have your ear right at my mouth, you will hear me at 100% volume. However, as you move away from my mouth, the sound volume will rapidly drop off according to the law of inverse squares. For example, if you just move away from my mouth 2 feet, then you put a 1 over the distance squared—in this case, 2 x 2 and you get ¼.

So just 2 feet away you will only hear me ¼ as loud. If you increase that distance to 8 feet, then you will only hear me 1/64th as loud. At 20 feet, you will only hear me 1/400th as loud. Couple this with your hearing loss, and this makes a dramatic difference.

Instead of having people vainly shouting at us, all we need to do is move closer together. For example, if you do a lot of your chatting in the living room, instead of arranging the seating the typical way—around the perimeter of the room, which means people are sitting far apart—clump the chairs close together and place them facing each other. Just moving the chairs closer together makes hearing ever so much easier.

Therefore, if you want to hear better, get close.

1.2 Background Noise Becomes a Problem with Increasing Distance

With increasing distance, more sounds come between you and the speaker—and because they are closer to you than you are from the speaker, you hear them better. As a result, they drown out the person you are talking to. This means any extraneous sounds from the audience such as coughing, papers crinkling, shifting in your seat, people talking, or any external sounds coming in through the windows or doors all make it more and more difficult to understand the speaker the further you are from him. Add to this the speech blocking effects of low-frequency sounds from the furnace, air-conditioning, fans, traffic noise, etc.

Wearing hearing aids doesn't really help in these cases, because with increasing distance you need to turn up your hearing aids more—and when you do that, your hearing aids pick up more and more background noise, and that interferes more and more with your ability to understand speech. If you are right here close to the speaker, you won't hear any of this background noise.

Therefore, to eliminate all this background noise, get close.

1.3 Speech Becomes Distorted with Increasing Distance

As speech sounds travel through the air, they are subject to distortion. For example, reverberation and reflections off hard surfaces in a room can distort speech. The closer you are to the speaker, the less you will hear this. If you are right here next to the speaker, you won't hear any distortion at all.

Therefore, to eliminate distortion, get close.

1.4 Speech Intelligence Drops with Increasing Distance

This is very important. Few people understand why this is so important. Did you know that the further you are from a speaker, the less intelligence there is in the speech sounds you hear. This means it becomes harder and harder to understand what the speaker is saying as the distance between you increases. Let me explain.

Most hard of hearing people have a **high**-frequency hearing loss. In an audiogram the low frequencies are at the left and the high frequencies are towards the right. A person with normal hearing has a line that goes across the top near the 0 dB line. A person with little hearing has a line near the bottom. However, most of you have a high frequency hearing loss so your audiogram looks sort of like a ski-hill on the left sloping down to the right. This indicates you don't hear too badly in the low frequencies, but your audiogram drops off dramatically in the higher frequencies.

Now follow this carefully. Most of the **volume** in speech is in the **low** frequencies, which you already hear not too badly—so you hear these low frequency sounds quite well.

However, most of the **intelligence** in speech is in the **softer high**-frequency sounds, which you don't hear much of at all.

Therefore, because you can still hear the low frequencies reasonably well, you can hear people talking, but because you can't hear the softer high frequencies well, if at all, you have great difficulty **understanding** what people are saying. You desperately need to hear those high-frequency sounds better in order to understand speech.

Now here's where it gets interesting.

Low-frequency sounds travel quite well through air so you can hear them at a greater distance. For example, the low-frequency component of my voice easily travels to the back of this room.

However, high frequency sounds attenuate quite fast in air so you can't hear them well from very far away. They rapidly drop out of the air with increasing distance. Picture the high-frequency sounds coming out of my mouth and falling in a pile on the floor close to my feet. The mid-frequency sounds travel farther and fall in a pile in the middle of the room, while the low-frequency sounds from my mouth zoom right to the back of the room.

What this all means is that the further your ears are from my mouth, the fewer high-frequency sounds you hear and consequently, the less you understand what I am saying because the sounds you need to understand speech are all laying here at my feet so to speak. They never reach your ears! So, if you want to hear all the intelligence in speech, you need to be right up here.

Therefore, in order to understand speech better, get close.

Getting Close—Here's How

There are two ways to get close.

One, get **physically** close. You do this by coming right up here and putting your ear close to my mouth. This works well in one-to-one situations, but won't work in groups.

Two, get close **electronically**. In groups you need assistive devices to help you get close electronically. (See chapter 6.)

If you don't remember anything else, remember that the single most important hearing loss coping strategy is simply this, **"Get close!"**

2. Fair Is Fair—Go to the Person

The second free and effective coping strategy I call "Fair is fair—go to the person". If you are not already close to the person you want to talk with, move closer. Do **not** call to us from another room and expect us to understand you. If you are in a different room, somebody has to move!

Here is the fair way to do it. If you want to talk to me (assuming I'm the hard of hearing person), it is **your** responsibility to **come** to where I am. Don't expect me to come running to you. You will save a lot of time and aggravation by putting aside your newspaper or jumping up for a minute and coming to me to effectively communicate your message. By the same token, if I want to talk to you (and you are in another room), I will come to you. Fair is fair.

It is not fair when the hard of hearing person calls/talks to the hearing person from another room, knowing they won't be able to hear the reply, and then expects the hearing person to come trotting out to where they are. First, **go to** the hearing person, **then** talk. This way you will be able to hear them when they reply.

The rule is very simple, whoever **initiates** the conversation has to go to the other person **before** beginning to talk.

3. Get the Person's Attention Before Beginning to Talk

Get our attention **before** you begin speaking to us. Here are three good ways you can do this. One, **approach** us in our **line of sight**. Two, **wave** your hand to attract our attention. Three, **touch** us lightly on the shoulder or arm. Often, just getting close is enough. It's hard to ignore a person that is standing nose to nose with you!

Next, give us time to focus on your face **before** you begin speaking or we will lose the first part of your conversation.

4. Talk Face-to-Face

Getting close, by itself isn't the whole answer. You need to face the person you are talking with unless, of course, you love repeating yourself! Position yourself so you can easily see our face and lips and so we can see yours.

This is most important. Notice that I did not say you **should** face us when talking to us. If you want to communicate effectively with us (and save yourself a lot of repetition and aggravation in the process), you **must** look at us. (Of course, this implies, too, that we are also looking at you! See text box.)

It is almost impossible for us to understand you if we cannot see your lips, facial expressions and gestures.

> **Andy & His Grandson**
>
> Andy's four-year-old grandson, Evan, had been instructed to always look at him when he wanted to talk to him because Andy is now severely hard of hearing. One day as Andy was going out the back door to do some chores on the farm, Evan called out from behind him, "Grandpa, can I come with you?"
>
> "Now, Evan," his mother admonished him, "you know that grandpa can't hear you when you are not looking at him."
>
> "But mommy," protested Evan staring at Andy's rapidly disappearing back, "I **am** looking at him!"

Therefore, we seldom, if ever, understand you if you are talking to us from another room, if you have your head buried in the newspaper or in the fridge, if you are walking away from us, or if you are calling us over a public address system.

5. Have Adequate Light

Almost all hard of hearing people speechread to some extent whether they realize it or not. We need lots of light in order to speechread and clearly see any gestures, facial expressions and body language. This becomes even more important as we age and our eyes need more light in order to see.

The direction from which the light comes is critical. Make sure the light is on your face if you are the speaker. In practical terms, this means do not stand in front of a bright light or window. This will put your face in a shadow. If your face is in the shadow, we cannot see you clearly enough to speechread. In addition, if the light source is behind you, it shines in our eyes and gives us both eyestrain and headaches. We have to squint into the light. It is decidedly difficult to speechread you when our eyes are narrowed to tiny slits!

Having your back to the light only works if you are talking with a hearing person. If there are two hard of hearing people, neither one can be backlit or the other one won't be able to speechread him clearly. The solution is to sit the chairs facing each other with the light coming from the side. That way both their faces are at least half in the light and make for passable speechreading.

In order to make our homes hard-of-hearing friendly, we may need to rearrange the lighting (or the seating) so that there is adequate light falling on everyone's faces but not in their eyes. This means that the traditional table lamps at eye level are out. Ceiling lights are the best as they are out of everyone's eyes and illuminate our faces. Unfortunately for us, ceiling lights are not in style in our homes today. The second choice is pole lamps with the lights high on the pole.

Another important thing to consider is the light coming in the windows. Yes, we want that light, but no, we don't want it in our eyes. As a result we mustn't arrange the living room furniture so that a chair or sofa is in front of the window. Anyone sitting there would be backlit by the outside light. To a person sitting across the room facing the window, that person's face would be in the shadow and very hard to speechread.

6. Cut Out Background Noise

Another enemy of understanding speech for hard of hearing people is background noise. Cut out as much noise as possible before you talk to us because we are bothered excessively by background sounds. You see, our ears cannot separate speech from background sounds like normal ears can. (People with normal hearing can hear speech clearly if it is just 6 dB above the background noise. For hard of hearing people, speech must be at least 15 dB, and often up to 25 dB, louder to achieve the same result.) In actual fact, we don't hear background sounds as such. When we wear hearing aids, **all** sounds are right there in the foreground competing with your voice.

Therefore, in order to understand you well, we need relative silence so your voice is the only thing we hear.

We generally cannot hear you above the noise of running water, rustling papers, other people talking, the TV, radio or stereo, a vacuum cleaner or similar sounds. Your words are buried in the noise. To a person with normal hearing, soothing background music may create the right mood, but to us it is just more obnoxious noise we have to try to hear you through.

When you want to chat with us, seek a quiet space with no background noise and few visual distractions.

One hundred years ago, houses were built with doors to each room. Now, we have open architecture and many times the living room, dining room and kitchen are all open to each other. The noise from one area travels freely to another area, and we have trouble hearing.

If you can, separate the noisy areas by shutting doors if you have them. Have children play downstairs or outside or in their bedrooms when you have hard of hearing guests in your home.

Turn off the TV, radio, and stereo as this just interferes with our ability to hear speech. The same is true for any other noisemakers in your house such as the dishwasher, washing machine, etc. These chores can wait until after the conversation is over.

If traffic or other outside noise is a problem, shut windows or doors on that side of the house or move to a quieter location in the house.

Another point: keep separate conversations in separate rooms. Two groups chatting in the same room make it almost impossible for us to understand much of anything. Move one group to another room. Both groups will then be able to chat to their hearts content without interfering with each other.

7. Avoid Miscommunication—Repeat Back What You Think You Heard—Especially Directions and Instructions

When we have hearing losses, a very real problem is the problem of miscommunication. Your spouse said one thing, and you heard another.

This happens because of several factors.

- One of course is our poor hearing.

- Two is poor discrimination—we don't understand what we are hearing—even when it is loud enough for us to hear it.

- Three, we may have our minds on other things.

- Four, we don't really understand what our spouse is driving at in the first place. This is a man/woman thing, not a hearing thing at all!

Therefore, we need to work to make sure what we are communicating is what our spouse is understanding.

In actual fact there are 4 possibilities how this works out in practice.

1. You **know** you heard correctly (and you **did**).

2. You're **not sure** you heard correctly (so you ask for a repeat to be sure).

3. You **know you didn't hear correctly** (or much at all) so you have to ask for a repeat.

4. You **know** you heard correctly but in actual fact, you got it wrong. You won't ask for clarification in this case because you **know** you got it right! (That's what makes this case so insidious—and where a lot of problems arise.)

The only way around this so that you know for sure if a hard of hearing person has the message right is to ask them to **repeat back** what they just heard. **Only what a hard of hearing person can repeat back to you is what he/she truly understood**. The onus is on you (the hearing person) to be sure that all the essential details are included.

Well, there you have it—seven effective and free coping strategies—get close, go to the speaker, face the speaker, get the person's attention, cut out background noise, have adequate light, and repeat back what was said.

Use them every day. They are so easy to put into practice—drill them into your head until they become second nature. If you follow these seven coping strategies, they will go a long way towards easing your frustrations and making conversing with people much easier and more enjoyable, and that makes it worth the extra effort.

Chapter 4

Hear with Your Eyes—the Art and Science of Speechreading

When I talk about speechreading, I am not talking about it as a stand-alone skill, but as an integral part of the overall strategy for successfully living with your hearing loss. You see, speechreading isn't perfect. Neither are our ears. Neither are hearing aids. Neither are assistive devices. That is why we need to use anything and everything at our disposal in order to help us understand as much speech as possible.

I am a "native" speechreader. By this I mean that speechreading was my first "language". Essentially, I've been speechreading from the day I was born. From as far back as I can remember, I knew that I had to look at people's faces if I was to have a hope of understanding what they were saying. Thus, what I'll be saying here comes from my 60+ years of speechreading every day, and from my experience teaching speechreading to others. I know how wonderful speechreading is, and at the same time, I well know its many limitations.

What Is Speechreading?

You probably know speechreading under its older term of lip reading. Technically, lip reading focuses on just the speaker's lips whereas speechreading takes in the whole body.

Speechreading is the ability to understand speech by using all the means available to us, including, but not limited to:

Observing the movement and appearance of the:

- lips
- jaw
- tongue
- teeth

Interpreting:

- facial expressions
- gestures
- body language

Analyzing what we know about:

- the structure of the language being spoken
- the topic being discussed

Using clues around you:

- situational clues
- environmental clues

What do I mean by situational and environmental clues? For example, if you are in the hospital, the conversation will be a lot different than if you are in a bank, or out boating, or in church, or at the scene of a traffic accident. Those are situational clues. Environmental clues are what is going on around you at the time. A fire alarm going off or a snowstorm outside would be environmental clues.

Therefore, in any situation you find yourself in, you can mentally prepare yourself for the kinds of things people likely will be talking about in these various situations. The more prepared you are, the easier you will find it to speechread people under those conditions.

Finally, speechreading, in its broadest sense, **includes anything at all that helps give a clue to what a person is saying** such as:

- using our residual hearing (this is very, very important)
- writing key words down

- fingerspelling
- simple signs

In the United Kingdom, they still use the term lip reading, but they really mean speechreading. I often use these two terms interchangeably, thus when I say lip reading, I really mean speechreading.

Speechreading is part art and part science, but it is actually much more art than science. That is why some people are better at it than others, just as some people are better artists or musicians than others.

Speechreading is not a particularly easy skill to acquire, neither is it particularly accurate—but it is **indispensable** nevertheless. Multitudes of hard of hearing people (myself included) speechread every day in order to effectively communicate with others.

Myths and Realities of Speechreading

You need to have realistic expectations of what speechreading can and cannot do for you, or you will be sadly disappointed. You all have seen the Hollywood version of speechreading. The hero somehow speechreads the villain—through binoculars—from half a mile away—in a blinding rainstorm—in the middle of the night. This is the Hollywood myth.

Here are a couple of other myths about speechreading.

Myth 1—All Hard of Hearing People Are Good Speechreaders

Not true. We are not all created equal in our ability to speechread. When we lose our hearing, our brains don't suddenly turn on a speechreading program that instantly makes us wonderful speechreaders.

It **is** true that almost all hard of hearing people speechread to some extent, whether they realize it or not, although the odd person just cannot seem to speechread at all. On the other hand, a few people are fantastic speechreaders. I know thousands and thousands of hard of hearing people, but I can count on the fingers of one hand the few incredible speechreaders I know. The vast majority of us fall somewhere in between these two extremes.

It is interesting (not fair, but interesting) that women, on the average, are much better speechreaders than men. This is just the way it is. We men have to struggle much more to speechread than women, yet it is we men that lose our hearing sooner, and have more severe hearing losses than women. I am a good speechreader, but there are women that make me look like I was still in speechreading kindergarten!

Myth 2—You Can Understand Everything When You Speechread

Again, not true. Speechreaders cannot understand everything you are saying. You may see this in the movies, but this is not true in real life.

English is not a particularly easy language to speechread. Some languages are easier (and some are even harder). The best estimates are that **30% to 35% of English sounds** can be speechread. In order for a sound to be easily speechread, it must be formed on the lips and/or in the front of the mouth.

Unfortunately for us, we form many English sounds in the middle of our mouths. Others come from the back of our mouths and even in our throats. These latter are absolutely impossible to speechread.

Furthermore, some speech sounds are totally invisible. For example, when I say the words "ear" and "hear" there is no visible difference. The "h" in "hear" is totally invisible.

Incidentally, in case you haven't noticed, **consonants** are formed by the **movements** of your mouth, whereas **vowels** are formed by the **shape** of your mouth. Often the vowel shapes are partially obscured by your mouth getting ready to form the next consonant.

As a result of all of this, a "perfect" speechreader theoretically only would be able to speechread about one third of what is said by observing the lips alone. They guess at the rest, taking into consideration their understanding of the structure of the spoken language, the body language of the speaker and what they know about the subject under discussion. Some people are remarkably good at this, but no one is perfect.

Homophenes

Another challenge in speechreading are words that sound different (if we could hear them), but look identical on a person's lips. We call such words homophenes.

For example, p, b and m are homophenes. Let me show you. When I say the words "**pat**", "**bat**" and "**mat**" you can hear the difference—but you cannot see any difference.

When we can't hear, we cannot tell these words apart. There are many homophones in English. For example, the words "**shoot**," "**shoes**," "**chews**," "**juice**," "**June**" and "**Jews**" all look exactly the same on a person's lips.

So do words as different as "**quiet**" and "**white**". So do the three words in the sentence, "**Buy my pie**."

Sometimes homophenes come in pairs—one voiceless and one voiced—but both have the identical mouth-shape. Examples of paired homophones include words such as "**few**" and "**view**", or "**pan**" and "**man**", or "**tad**" and "**dad**", or "**calf**" and "**gaff**".

And who would have thought that words as different as "**ship**" and the man's name "**Jim**" would look identical on a person's lips.

In such cases, there is no way you can tell what word was spoken by lip reading alone. You either need some hearing, or know the context, so you can figure out what the word must have been.

Some words become homophenes because the first letter in the word is totally invisible. For example, in the case of "**oat**", "**coat**" and "**goat**", the "c" and the "g" are totally invisible. The same is true in with the words "**at**", "**cat**" and "**hat**". Here, the "c" and the "h" are totally invisible. Thus when a person says "coat" or "goat", we only see the word "oat", and when a person says "cat" or "hat", all we see is the word "at".

The Secret to Good Speechreading

The real secret to effective speechreading is to combine speechreading with your **residual hearing**. And of course, your residual hearing is much better if you wear hearing aids and/or use assistive listening devices.

One study showed that by listening only, hard of hearing people could understand about 24% of speech. By speechreading alone, these same people only understood 12%, which seems to indicate that speechreading is pretty much a waste of time, doesn't it? But hang on for a second. By combining both residual hearing and speechreading, they understood, not the expected 36%, but a whopping 79% of speech. See how much speechreading really helps when you have some residual hearing?

My friend BJ found that she could speechread 34% without her hearing aids. With her hearing aids, but not speechreading, she could get 16%. However, when she combined speechreading with her residual hearing, she understood 88% (not just the expected 50%).

Researchers at the University of Manchester found similarly impressive results when hard of hearing people wore hearing aids and speechread at the same time. In one study, hard of hearing people just using their residual hearing understood 21% of speech. If they combined their residual hearing with either a hearing aid or with speechreading, they could understand 64% of speech. This is a significant improvement. However, if they used their residual hearing and both hearing aids and speechreading, their speech comprehension soared to 90%. This is why speechreading is so important if you want to successfully live with your hearing loss.

One of the reasons why combining residual hearing and speechreading is so effective is because most people have a high-frequency hearing loss. Thus they don't hear the higher-pitched consonants, but they do hear the lower-pitched vowel sounds. Now follow this. Because the consonants are formed by mouth movements, we can often "see" these sounds. At the same time, the harder-to-distinguish vowel sounds are louder, and because most have quite good low-frequency hearing, they hear the vowels.

This combination of hearing the vowels and seeing the consonants together gives us pretty good comprehension as the above results attest.

Speechreading Basics

Here's a few things you should know about speechreading.

You Need Reasonable Vision

People hear and understand better when they can clearly see the speaker. In fact, the House Ear Institute a few years ago released a paper entitled **"You Can Hear Better with Your Glasses On"**. This was just an interesting way of saying that all people, whether hearing or hard of hearing, speechread to some extent, especially when listening conditions are less than ideal.

Always Watch the Person Speaking

The one bad habit that absolutely guarantees that you will fail at speechreading is **not watching the speaker's face at all times**.

When they are concentrating in a difficult hearing situation, often hearing people either stare at the floor or the ceiling, or shut their eyes. This is the worst habit that people who lose their hearing later in life have to break. You just cannot speechread when you are not staring at the person speaking. I have actually seen a student speechreading instructor staring at the floor deep in concentration—straining to hear—but little good it did him as the instructor was silently mouthing the words!

Know the Subject and the Context

In order for speechreading to be effective, we have to know both the subject being discussed and its context. So often we are told to get the meaning from the context, but if we don't know the subject or the context, we are lost.

One good way to know the subject is to keep up to date on what is going on in the media and around you. That way you will be knowledgeable about likely subjects of conversation. This gives you a big advantage in speechreading.

When we know both the subject and the context, we then try to anticipate what the person is going to say. This helps us speechread much better. However, we still have to carefully watch the speaker's mouth to be sure he says what we think he is going to say. If we slack off, we can inadvertently end up in left field!

Incidentally, because names and short remarks don't have any context, we often don't catch them. Names could be as simple of Joe Brown, or harder like Makayla Sternodova.

Slower Is Better

Another thing you should know about speechreading is that during normal speech, a person make approximately 13 to 15 speech movements per second. However, our eyes can only pick up and our brains process 8 or 9 of these movements each second. Thus, if a person is talking at a normal rate, we will miss between one quarter and one half of what he says just because our brains can't keep up. Therefore, if you are having trouble speechreading someone, ask the person to slow down. You'll find it really helps your comprehension. Another benefit of speaking more slowly is that the speaker then typically moves his lips more, and that makes speechreading even easier.

Speechreading Is Tiring

A downside of speechreading, and one that is not obvious, is that the enormous concentration required in speechreading is exhausting. This is especially true with someone who is hard to speechread in the first place. When speechreading, your eyes must follow every lip movement, every facial expression, every gesture, then your brain has to take what your eyes saw, what little your ears heard, what you already know about the structure of the

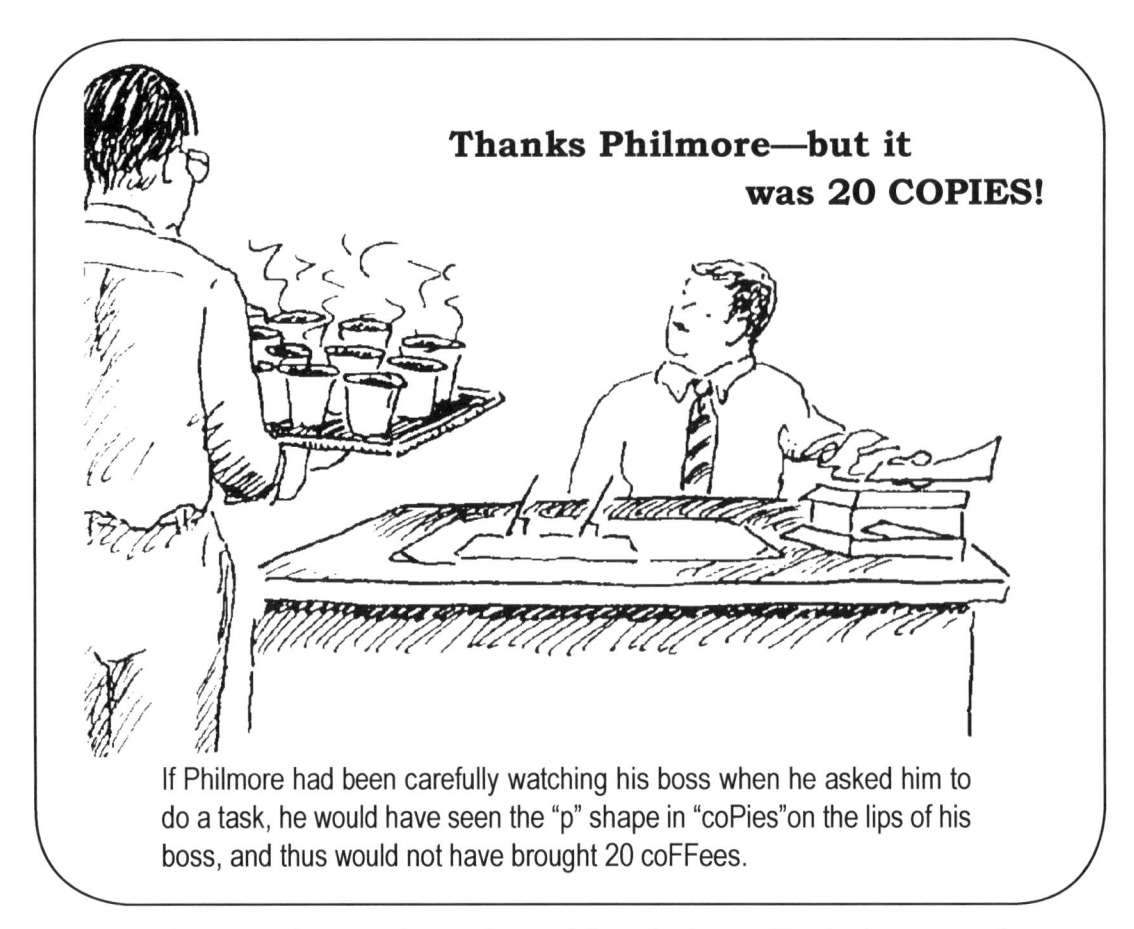

> **Thanks Philmore—but it was 20 COPIES!**
>
> If Philmore had been carefully watching his boss when he asked him to do a task, he would have seen the "p" shape in "coPies" on the lips of his boss, and thus would not have brought 20 coFFees.

language, what you know about the subject being talked about, and try to put this together while at the same time substituting various homophenes to find the right match, and hopefully coming up with a meaningful message.

As you can imagine, this takes a lot of brainpower. I've heard that our brains have to work five times as hard to understand speech as do the brains of people with normal hearing. No wonder speechreading makes us tired! We cannot relax our eyes for even a split second and have a nice easy conversation like people with normal hearing can.

Some People Are Easy to Speechread, Some Aren't

Finally, some people are very easy to speechread. They are a pleasure to talk to. Unfortunately, when you do well speechreading one person, your family/friends/co-workers might think that you can do that with anyone. This is just not true.

At the same time, be aware that a small proportion of the population move their lips in such a way that it is absolutely impossible to speechread even one word they say. Don't beat yourself up when you can't speechread them. It's definitely not your fault.

There is one sportscaster on the TV who is absolutely impossible to speechread. I have tried and tried, but have never been able to even speechread a single syllable he speaks. Even the Muppets are easier to speechread than him!

In spite of its many shortcomings, I for one would never want to be without speechreading. It's that important!

If you want to learn to speechread better, try to find a speechreading class nearby. If there are no speechreading classes nearby, all is not lost. You can order a wonderful speechreading CD program from the Center for Hearing Loss Help website at http://www.hearinglosshelp.com/products/seeinghearingspeech.htm. This CD will help you learn speechreading in the privacy of your own home using your computer.

Chapter 5

Hearing Aids—Here's What You Need to Know about Them

Too often, people think that wearing hearing aids is the whole answer to hearing loss. When they find out that hearing aids don't return hearing to normal, they are sorely disappointed and tell everyone that hearing aids don't work. In truth, hearing aids do work, but they are only part of the solution.

Wearing hearing aids is only one of the five parts to successfully coping with your hearing loss. I want to emphasize again that hearing aids by themselves are just not enough. You also have to speechread, use effective coping strategies, use assistive devices when appropriate and be problem-focused in regards to your hearing needs. When you do all of these, you will find that your hearing aids work ever so much better!

Like their name implies, hearing aids are aids to hearing, not cures for hearing loss. They do not restore your hearing to normal, especially if you have a more severe hearing loss.

Getting the right hearing aids for your hearing loss, lifestyle and pocketbook is often both stressful and confusing, especially if you are buying your first set of hearing aids. The good news is that in this chapter you will learn the key things you need to know about hearing aids before you spend even a single cent!

1. Have the Proper Expectations of What Hearing Aids Can and Cannot Do for You

It is most important that you have the proper expectations of what hearing aids can and cannot do for you. I can't stress this enough. Here are some points to help you form proper expectations of what your hearing aids can do for you.

1.1 Hearing aids will not restore your hearing to normal. You will still be hard of hearing to some degree. Furthermore, the sounds from your hearing aids will not be the same as sounds from your natural ears, although these sounds may be near-normal. At the very least, understanding speech should be better than without wearing hearing aids, but you will still not hear speech perfectly. Therefore, after spending the big bucks on hearing aids, don't be dismayed when you find that your audiologist failed to mention that you will still need to get some assistive devices, you will still need to speechread, and you will still need to use various other coping strategies, particularly if listening conditions are less than ideal, or if you have a more severe hearing loss.

1.2 Hearing aids only correct your hearing loss to about half of what it was before. Hearing aids do not bring you back up to normal, especially if you have a more severe loss. Therefore, expect to hear better than before. Don't expect normal hearing.

1.3 Hearing aids work best in quiet situations. The more noise there is around you, the less effective your hearing aids will be.

1.4 Hearing aids work best when you are close to the speaker—no more than 6 to 10 feet away. The greater the distance you are from the speaker, the less effective your hearing aids will become.

1.5 Since both noise and distance are enemies of hearing aids, in these situations you need to combine your hearing aids with assistive technology in order to hear effectively. Combining hearing aids with assistive devices can turn your hearing aids into awesome hearing devices. If you do this, you will swear by them. If you don't, you may swear at them.

Let me emphasize it again—always keep in mind that hearing aids are not the whole answer. If you remember this, and use all the coping strategies covered in this book, you will probably be delighted with your hearing aids.

2. How Many Hearing Aids Do You Need?

People often ask, "Do I need two hearing aids, or is wearing one good enough?" The answer is simple. How many ears did God give you? God gave us two ears for a reason—not because He had a bunch of ears left over from the time of creation that He wanted to use up. If you have a hearing loss in both ears, then you need to wear two hearing aids.

There are a number of advantages to wearing two hearing aids. Here are some of them.

2.1 You will understand much more of what you hear with two hearing aids than you would with just one. This is because optimum hearing and sound processing occurs when you use both ears. In addition, both sides of your brain work differently. Thus, you need both ears working together in what is called "auditory synergy" in order to get the maximum benefit from what you hear.

2.2 Hearing will be easier and consequently less tiring because you won't have to strain as much.

2.3 You can better tell where sound is coming from. With one hearing aid, you just hear the sound inside your head without any reference to direction, so you won't be able to tell who is speaking, or where a warning sound is coming from. Thus, wearing two hearing aids is safer. Also, if the battery in one hearing aid dies or the hearing aid itself dies, you will still have your other hearing aid to help you hear in the meantime.

2.4 With two hearing aids, you hear from both sides of your head. With only one aid, you may apparently be "rudely" ignoring a person on your deaf side. If you are totally deaf in one ear, there are special CROS/Bi-CROS aids (CROS stands for "Contralateral Routing Of Sound") that take the sound from your deaf side and pipe it to your opposite ear. In this way. you can still hear sounds from your deaf side, but you hear them in your good ear. (Note: CROS aids are for people with one normally-hearing ear and one deaf ear. Bi-CROS aids are for people with one hard of hearing ear and one deaf ear.)

2.5 Hearing and understanding speech in noise is better and easier. In fact, you only need half the volume for the same degree of understanding when you wear two hearing aids instead of just one. Because of this, the background noise won't be as loud either. This cuts down on the number of "noise" headaches you may experience.

There are two exceptions to the rule of wearing two hearing aids. The first one is obvious. If one ear can't hear anything in the first place, then wearing a normal hearing aid (not a CROS or Bi-CROS aid) in that ear is useless.

The second exception to the two-hearing-aid rule is if one ear hears completely garbled sound (poor discrimination) and the other ear has reasonably good discrimination. In this case, wearing a hearing aid in the garbled ear makes it very difficult for your brain to filter out the garbage in order to understand speech from your better ear. Therefore, if wearing two hearing aids reduces your comprehension, then only wear a hearing aid in your better ear, or wear a Bi-CROS aid.

3. Becoming Friends with Your New Hearing Aids

One of the places many people go wrong is right at the beginning when they get new hearing aids. Here's a typical scenario.

The big day arrives. You are excited, and you should be. You are going to hear again today! Today you will receive your brand new hearing aids. Your audiologist carefully fits and adjusts them to your own special needs. She tests you with them to be sure you hear as well as possible.

You are thrilled as you leave the building and step out into the street. Suddenly a horrible roar assaults your ears. You are shocked right out of your socks! You don't ever remember that traffic was this noisy. You can't stand the awful racket. Quickly you reach up and yank your hearing aids out of your ears and stuff them into your pocket. And your dream of hearing again is shattered.

What went wrong? Just this—you expected instant success. It doesn't work that way. So the question becomes, "How do I best learn to wear my new hearing aids?" Here are four tips.

3.1 You need to give your brain time to adjust. Therefore, slowly adjust to wearing your new hearing aids. You must be patient. It can take 60 to 90 days or more for your brain to adjust to new hearing aids.

3.2 Wear your hearing aids at home (or other quiet place) to start with. You are not ready to deal with louder sounds right at the outset.

3.3 Begin wearing your hearing aids maybe only half an hour or an hour a day and increase the time each day by half an hour or an hour until you are wearing them all the time. The worse your hearing loss is when you get new hearing aids, the more critical this is. Set a schedule that works for you. While your brain is getting used to the louder sounds, your ear canals are getting used to having ear molds in them.

3.4 After you are comfortable wearing your hearing aids in relatively quiet places for several hours at a time, then slowly graduate to noisier situations.

If you follow these four key steps, the day will come when you will actually feel undressed unless you are wearing your hearing aids. Finally, one day the realization will hit you that you and your hearing aids have indeed become close friends, but it does take time.

4. Which Hearing Aid Is the Best?

Now comes the perennial question, "Which is the best hearing aid?" That's like asking, "Which is the best car?" Some people say a Rolls Royce is the best. It may be the most elegant car, but is it the best car? Young guys don't want a Rolls; they want a $750,000.00 Ferrari. It beats the Rolls Royce hands down as a high-performance sports car, but is a Ferrari the best car? Outdoorsmen say, "Get a Hummer". It's the best. Then you can go way back in the hills—places a Rolls or a Ferrari can't go because the track is too rough for them.

It's the same with hearing aids. There are elegant hearing aids, there are sexy sports model hearing aids and there are rough and ready workhorses. Each is designed for a given situation (besides helping you hear better).

Therefore, the real question you should be asking is not "Which is the best hearing aid?" but, "Which is the best hearing aid **for me**?" You see, the best hearing aid for you depends on your specific needs. For example, do you need to hear while you are swimming underwater? If so, the hearing aid for you is the Rion Dolphin because it is totally waterproof.

If you want to be able to pair your hearing aids with your bluetooth cell phone and plug your iPod directly into your hearing aids so you can hear both of these devices in both ears, then maybe you need to look at a hearing aids such as Oticon's Epoq. But if you want to listen to your MP3 player in true stereo via your hearing aids, then you'll need a hearing aid like the Phonak Exelia.

If you can only hear low frequency sounds (have no high frequency hearing left) then you might find a frequency-shifting hearing aid such as Sonovation's ImpaCt fits your specific hearing needs.

In truth, there are many factors to consider when getting a new hearing aid. Some of them are subjective, so only you can make the decision, while others are objective, and your audiologist can choose those for you. For example, your audiologist can tell you which aids have enough power for your hearing loss, but only you can determine if the sound produced by these aids seems "good" to you. Furthermore, only you know which features are important to you. Therefore, the best hearing aid for you is the one that has the power, clarity and features you need.

Once you've narrowed your choices down to a short list of hearing aids that have the features you want, and the power and type that your audiologist knows you need, how do you make your final choice?

The surprising answer is that when it comes right down to it, your satisfaction with any of these hearing aids on your short list will depend, not so much on a specific hearing aid, but on the skills of the person programming it to your specific needs.

Therefore, ultimately you want to purchase a hearing aid that your audiologist has had lots of experience successfully programming, and also knows how to program it to fit your specific hearing needs. This is expecially important if you have an unusual hearing loss such as I have.

Dr. Mark Ross, a man I highly respect because of his common-sense understanding of hearing loss, both as a highly-regarded audiologist, and also as a hard of hearing person, wrote an article called "Revisiting the Perennial Question: What is the 'Best' Hearing Aid". You can read it in the January/February 2009 issue of Hearing Loss magazine put out by the Hearing Loss Association of America (HLAA), or you can read this article on their website at http://www.hearingloss.org/magazine/2009JanFeb/HLMJanFeb09BestHearingAid.pdf.

5. A Dozen Tips to Help You When Buying New Hearing Aids

Here are a number of tips to help you avoid being "taken in" when you are considering getting new hearing aids.

5.1 Get the best hearing aids for you. Don't worry about all the fancy bells and whistles. Get hearing aids that fit your lifestyle—ones that will let you hear when and where you most need to. In other words buy hearing aids with the features you will actually use.

5.2 Do your homework regarding hearing aids. If you can't name and describe possible benefits for at least 3 features of hearing aids, then you need to do more homework. At the very least, you should know the benefits of directional microphones, T-coils (telecoils) and the various kinds of ear molds—vented ear molds, open-fitted ear molds and Receiver-in-the-Ear (RITE) styles. Learn which features and styles of hearing aids are best for your own lifestyle and hearing loss. For example, if you have arthritic fingers, then maybe automatic aids will be better for you. If you have limited shoulder mobility, then having a remote control will be better for you than reaching up to your ears to adjust your hearing aids. If you have poor vision, then you certainly don't want the smallest model, or you'll never find it again when you put it down!

5.3 Don't be taken in by hype, or by glitzy ads, or by high pressure salesmen. For example, the bigger and more frequent the advertisement, the more cautious you should be. The more the ad promises, the less you should be willing to believe it. Furthermore, never buy a hearing aid that is offered at a "special price" if you must decide immediately. That is just high-pressure tactics to separate you from your money.

5.4 Make sure you know the terms of the trial period. By law, you have a 30 day trial period. (Some places will give you 45 or 60 days, but 30 days is the minimum allowed.) You can return your hearing aids within this time and exchange them for different models or get a refund. Generally there is a return fee. Did you know this? Find out what the return fee is before you sign on the dotted line. Typically fees range from $50 to $300 (or roughly around 10% of the total price of each hearing aid). In my opinion, all you really should have to pay for is the hearing evaluation and ear mold. Fortunately, a few hearing aid dispensers do not charge you this return fee.

5.5 Shop around to get a good price. Prices can vary as much as $1,000 for a given hearing aid, so it can really be worth your while to ask around.

5.6 Get T-coils (sometimes called telecoils or audiocoils). Ask your hearing aid dispenser whether the hearing aid he recommends has a T-coil. If he says you don't need one, walk out. (Anyone that ignorant about the benefits of t-coils shouldn't be selling hearing aids in the first place!) In my opinion, if the hearing aids you are considering don't have t-coils, don't buy them. T-coils are that useful! With T-coils you can couple your hearing aids to wonderful assistive devices such as room loops, FM systems and personal amplifiers with special microphones.

5.7 Hearing aids don't last forever. Be prepared to spend big bucks every few years. Depending on the models you choose, you may have to replace them every 3 to 5 years. Behind-the-Ear (BTE) hearing aids can last as long as 10 to 14 years if you are careful. In-the-ear (ITE) hearing aids do not last as long as BTE or Over-the-Ear (OTE) hearing aids—a good reason to get BTE/OTE hearing aids.

5.8 Expect to return for adjustments several times—maybe up to 10 times or more—in the first few weeks. Fitting hearing aids is both art and science. The fitting algorithms hearing aid manufacturers use only take into consideration the science part. The audiologist's personal experience is needed to supply the human factor (the art part).

5.9 Don't concern yourself about small size, cosmetic appeal or invisibility. People that purchase tiny, invisible hearing aids are often sorry when they find out just how limited these hearing aids are. Poor hearing in itself is much more "visible" than any hearing aids you might wear! Note this well: if the vendor's primary selling point is that the hearing aid is invisible, be very suspicious. If invisibility is your primary concern, then examine your motives. Hearing better is the real reason to buy a hearing aid, not invisibility!

5.10 Buy hearing aids with lots of reserve power. You should be running your hearing aids about half their capacity. That way, if your hearing continues to drop, you don't need to buy new hearing aids, you just turn up the volume. This can save you a lot of money in the long run.

5.11 Ask if they do "real ear" testing. "Real ear" testing is very important. It proves whether your hearing aids are doing what they are supposed to be doing. With "real ear" testing, the audiologist puts a tiny microphone into your ear canal, then inserts your hearing aid. Next, she compares what the hearing aid is supposed to be putting out with what the tiny microphone actually picks up. If the microphone shows the hearing aid is hitting the target graph, then the hearing aid is adjusted properly for your hearing loss. If it's not, it needs to be reprogrammed or a different hearing aid used. Without real ear testing, there is no objective way to know whether a hearing aid is really set properly for your hearing loss or not.

5.12 Have manual overrides for automatic features. Automatic hearing aids sound wonderful—let the hearing aid make all the adjustments for you. The problem is that your hearing aids don't know exactly what you like. Take volume for instance. Sometimes the sound may be too loud or too soft for you. If the volume is controlled automatically, you can't adjust it. Thus, if sounds are too loud for you in a noisy restaurant, for example, your only choices are to tough it out or leave. If you have

Chapter 5: Hearing Aids—Here's What You Need to Know

a manual volume override, then you can adjust the volume yourself at that point. The same is true for T-coils. Automatic T-coils are great if you use the telephone a lot, but they won't automatically switch for neckloops or room loops. For example, if you don't have a manual override, you won't be able to use loop systems to listen to your TV at home. I believe so much in having manual overrides for automatic features that I won't consider a hearing aid without manual overrides. To me they are that important!

Hearing aid technology is changing so fast, that it is almost impossible to keep up with all the changes. Therefore, when the time comes to buy new hearing aids, you need to do your own research on the current features, then decide what features you want in your "ideal" hearing aids. Don't leave those decisions up to your audiologist or hearing aid dispenser. You are the one that will be wearing them, so get the hearing aids that give you the best listening experiences possible. At the same time don't forget the skills of your audiologist and other human factors.

In closing, I want to re-emphasize four of these key points. I'm quoting some snippets here from one hearing professional.

1. "The best chance for success is making sure you have realistic expectations and a good rehabilitation program."

2. "Hearing aids do not restore hearing. Anyone who believes that will be disappointed."

3. "People make the basic assumption that the different hearing aid brands actually matter. Although the hearing aid manufacturers are actively promoting this idea, it usually is not the case."

4. "The real difference in hearing success is how well you work with the person who is fitting your hearing aids. Different people have different needs. Thus you need to find someone with the right skill set for your particular needs."

When you do this, you too will be successful in your quest for a hearing aid that best meets your needs.

Chapter 6

Assistive Technology—Turn Your Hearing Aids into Awesome Hearing Devices

Hard of hearing people often lament, "Hearing aids don't work well for me, particularly in noisy places such as while driving in the car or talking in noisy restaurants." They then ask, "What can I do in order to hear my spouse under such conditions? Being unable to communicate freely is putting a strain on our marriage. Can you help me?"

The answer is, "You bet I can!"

Unfortunately, when people lose their hearing, they are typically told to get hearing aids, as if hearing aids were the whole answer to hearing loss. However, when you are in difficult listening situations such as in noisy places, or are at some distance from the speaker, your expensive hearing aids can be almost useless! As a result, you may become disillusioned with your hearing aids.

You see, noise and distance are two enemies of hearing aids. That's the bad news. The good news is that assistive devices exist to conquer these two enemies. They have two main purposes in life; first, to effectively reduce the distance between you and the person to whom you are listening; and second, to reduce background noise so you can hear as clearly as your damaged ears allow you to hear.

Generally, you can use assistive devices with, or without, your hearing aids—but properly teamed up with your hearing aids, they can make an awesome combination, even in poor listening environments!

Benefits of Assistive Listening Devices

In Chapter 3, I wrote that the single most effective hearing loss coping strategy was "get close". Even if you can't get close physically, you can still get close electronically. You get close electronically by having the microphone of an assistive device close to the speaker's mouth, and through various means piping the sound directly into your ears or your hearing aids without these sounds having to travel though the air.

When you do this, two wonderful things happen.

You Get Unbelievable Clarity

First, when you use assistive devices properly, you get unbelievable clarity of speech. Consequently your understanding soars. Why won't your expensive hearing aids do the same as these relatively cheap assistive devices? Glad you asked. Remember, in Chapter 3 I explained how high-frequency sounds rapidly drop out of the air with increasing distance so few reach your ears. Remember, also, I said that it was these same high-frequency sounds that give speech much of its intelligence and clarity?

Think about it. If you are sitting at some distance from the speaker, and wearing your hearing aids, where are your hearing aids' microphones? You got it—right there on the top of your ears and far from the speaker's mouth.

Since the high-frequency sounds that pour forth from the speaker's mouth land on the floor somewhere in front of him (figuratively speaking), obviously they **never** reach your hearing aids' microphones. If they never reach your hearing aids microphones, you never will hear these sounds. It's not the fault of your hearing aids. It's the fault of the increasing distance from the speaker.

In contrast, if the speaker is wearing a microphone, the high-frequency sounds only travel in the air (as sound waves) the few inches between the speaker's mouth and the microphone. The result is that the microphone captures **all** the high-frequency sounds before they (figuratively) fall on the floor in front of the speaker.

From then on, these sounds never travel through the air as sound waves, but in some other form—either radio waves (FM systems), or light waves (infrared systems), or as a varying magnetic field (loop systems) or though a wire (personal amplifiers). As a result, all the clarity and intelligence of the speaker's voice reaches your ears, and you hear beautiful, clear sound, or at least as beautiful and clear a sound as your faulty ears permit you to hear.

Chapter 6: Assistive Technology

This is why, if you are at any distance from a speaker, you **need** to supplement your hearing aids with appropriate assistive devices.

Let me illustrate just how effective assistive devices can be. I'm the coordinator of the Adams/York chapter of the Hearing Loss Association of America (HLAA) in southern Pennsylvania. We loop our meeting room.

At one meeting, I was sitting in the first row right in front of the speaker—about 10 feet away. With my hearing aids in the microphone setting, and by speechreading at the same time, I could understand the speaker, but I had to pay attention. When I switched my hearing aids to their t-coils, suddenly the speaker's voice was wonderfully clear—just like he was talking into both of my ears at the same time—which, in effect, he was. His speech was so clear that I could look away and still easily understand him. (I didn't have to rely so much on my speechreading skills as I would have had to otherwise.)

Just to prove to myself how effective room loops are, I got up and walked to the back of the room. With my hearing aids back in their microphone mode, I really had to strain to understand the speaker. (As you can appreciate, speechreading isn't all the great from 30 feet away!) All the crispness had gone out of his voice. He sounded very bassy. However, when I switched my t-coils on again—wow! The speaker's voice instantly became clear and crisp—just like he was talking right into both of my ears again. The sound I was hearing was just as clear and crisp at the back of the room as it was at the front.

This is how dramatic the difference in understanding speech can be when you get electronically close via your hearing aids and assistive devices.

Background Noise All But Disappears

The second benefit of assistive devices is that they reduce or eliminate all background noise. When you try to hear in noise, often your expensive hearing aids are almost useless. All the noise between you and the speaker gets amplified along with the speaker's voice. The result is that you have trouble understanding much of anything.

Here is an example. Picture this. You have your hearing aids on and are sitting in your living room trying to listen to your favorite TV program. There is only one problem. You are babysitting your grandkids, and they are playing and laughing and talking and sometimes fighting and shrieking right at your feet. Your hearing aids are picking up all their racket. As a result, you cannot understand your TV program. Your expensive hearing aids do **nothing** for you in this situation.

Now picture this same scenario, but this time using an appropriate assistive device. The grandkids are making just as much racket by your feet as before—but you sit there oblivious to their shrieks as you enjoy your favorite program—hearing it clearly without any interference. The difference is like night and day. That can be **your** experience when you couple the **correct** assistive device to your hearing aids. Sounds incredible, doesn't it?—but once you've tried it, you'll know it's true!

You see, assistive devices, when properly used, cut out most background noise in one of two ways. In the above example, the assistive device was plugged directly into the sound source (TV) totally eliminating the microphone so it couldn't pick up any background noise. (You listen via the t-coils in your hearing aids, not via their microphones.)

In those situations when a microphone **is** used, the microphone is located much, much closer to the speaker's mouth than it is to the surrounding background noise. This effectively eliminates most of the background sounds.

For example, you are in a meeting and the people around you are coughing, talking, clinking dishes and rustling papers. Your hearing aids' microphones are picking up all these extraneous sounds. Consequently, you are having trouble understanding the speaker. However, with properly-used assistive devices, you will **only** hear the sounds going into the speaker's microphone, not the disturbing noise around you, because you have cut out your hearing aids' microphones and are now listening via their t-coils.

These devices really do work! Here are some real-life examples using one of my favorite assistive devices, a personal amplifier called the PockeTalker.

When my first wife and I would go driving, she'd often look out the side window. One day she exclaimed, "Wow look at that enormous bull elk!" Of course I couldn't hear her and said "What?" Still looking out the side window, she repeated, "Look at that elk!"

Again, but a little louder, I said, "What?" By that time we were past the elk. She turned to me and said, "Boy you missed seeing a big elk back there!" Exasperated, I retorted, "Why didn't you tell me?" (As you can see, we had some very intelligent conversations!) That's often the case when one spouse can't hear much.

Today, when my wife and I go driving, I simply clip my trusty lapel microphone to her sweater, plug it into my PockeTalker, and either plug in my ear buds (if I'm not wearing my hearing aids), or plug in a neckloop and switch my hearing aids to their t-coils. The difference is like night and day.

Now, I hear my wife clearly. She can talk all she wants without me having to ask for many repeats. It's wonderful!

We use this same arrangement in noisy restaurants. For example, one time we were in a Steakhouse restaurant. Although we were sitting well away from the bar where a TV was showing a football game, even with my hearing aids on, I couldn't hear my wife through all the racket from the boisterous patrons at the bar whenever someone made a good play or scored a touchdown!

What did I do? I whipped out my PockeTalker, clipped my lapel microphone to my wife's sweater, put on my neckloop and switched to t-coil mode. Instantly, the racket subsided, and I now could clearly hear my wife.

Another example: when I attend conventions, especially when I'm in the exhibit halls, it is very noisy. Even with my hearing aids on, I still constantly have to speechread in order to understand anything at all—not to mention getting headaches from all the racket.

Now, I simply haul out of my PockeTalker, but in these situations I plug in my super-directional microphone. I hold it down at my waist and aim at the face of the person I am talking to. (You don't have to stuff the microphone right in the person's face.)

If you haven't experienced it, you won't believe the difference! Instead of drowning in noise, I now hear beautiful, clear speech in both my ears. The difference is that dramatic!

This is what assistive devices do for me. They can do the same for you.

Types of Assistive Listening Devices

By now you are likely itching to learn more about these wonderful assistive devices.

There are a number of different technologies used in assistive devices in order to get the sound from the speaker's mouth to your ears. However, be aware that no technology gives significantly better sound than any other—they all do the same thing—deliver beautiful, clear sound directly to your ears.

Therefore, choose your assistive devices, not based on any given technology, but based on your specific needs, what you can afford, what devices are available to you, and what works best in the particular listening situation you are in.

Here are the five basic assistive technologies in current use today. They are:

- Personal amplifiers
- FM systems
- Infra-red systems
- Induction loop systems
- Bluetooth systems

Here's a brief look at each of these so you can see why you might choose one over another in any given situation.

1. Personal Amplifiers

Typically you would use a personal amplifier such as the PockeTalker when you are close to the person speaking and are not moving around, for example, listening to your spouse or friend when riding in a car, or conversing in a noisy restaurant. You clip a lapel microphone to the person with whom you are conversing, plug it into your personal amplifier, plug in a neckloop (or Music Links) and listen to your partner via the t-coils in your hearing aids. This cuts out much of the background noise.

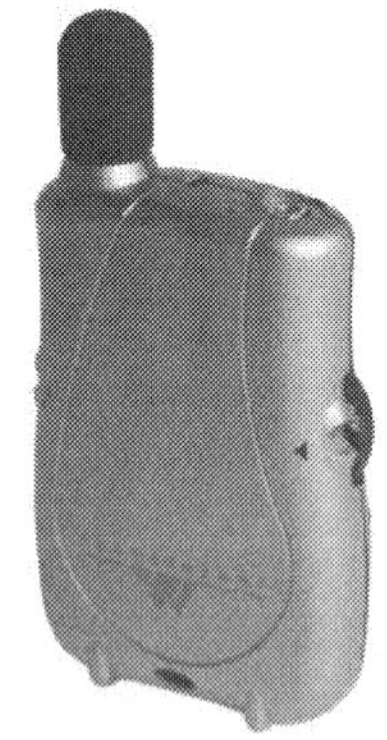

If you want to be able to walk around, then just substitute the lapel microphone with the super-directional hand-held microphone, and aim it at the person with whom you are talking.

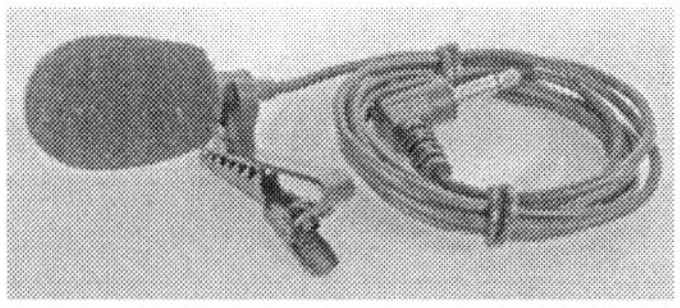

PockeTalker Ultra

Lapel Microphone

The downside of the lapel microphone arrangement is that you are wired together and thus are not free to move around. However, in situations where you are both sitting down this is not a problem. You can also use these devices to listen to your TV by attaching the microphone of your assistive device near the TV's speaker and running a microphone extension cord across the room to your PockeTalker. You can do the same if the person you are talking to is sitting on

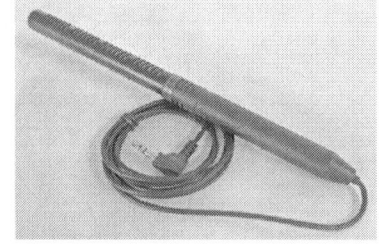

Super-directional Hand-held Microphone

the other side of the room. This is typically the cheapest way to go. The cost is around $200.00 with the lapel microphone.

To learn more of the benefits of using a personal amplifier such as the PockeTalker, read my article "Hear In Noise? You Bet You Can! Here's How" (http://www.hearinglosshelp.com/articles/hearinnoise.htm). You can see pictures and the features of the PockeTalker and the various microphones I use (and order them for yourself) at http://www.hearinglosshelp.com/products/pocketalker.htm.

2. FM Systems

FM systems (FM stands for "frequency modulation") use radio waves to transmit the sound from the speaker's mouth to your ears. Because there are no wires connecting you to the speaker, you are free to move around, or sit at some distance from the speaker. For example, you can typically be up to 150 feet away from the speaker and still hear just as well as if the person was talking directly into both of your ears. Of course, this requires the person speaking to cooperate and use/wear your wireless FM microphone/transmitter.

You can use FM systems even if you have to go into an adjacent room, or if you are outside walking or riding your bicycle with a friend. You will hear your friend's voice beautifully clear in your ears as long as you stay within 150 feet of each other.

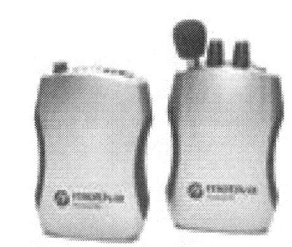

Motiva PFM 360 Personal FM System (Transmitter - left, Receiver - right)

One drawback of FM systems is that they tend to be relatively expensive—in the neighborhood of $700.00 and up, although a few are much cheaper—around $200.00. You can see a good personal FM system, which doubles as a PockeTalker on the Center's website at http://www.hearinglosshelp.com/products.htm#pfm360.

3. Infrared Systems

Infrared systems are similar to FM systems, except they use light waves instead of radio waves to transmit the sound. Typically, infrared systems are used in meeting halls/theaters and for watching TV.

However, infrared systems are not as versatile as FM systems because of two things. First, you cannot use them outside or in a room with a lot of sunlight streaming in—as the infrared component of the sun's rays causes horrible interference. So too, do many flat-screen plasma TVs. Second, light waves travel in straight lines. Thus your infrared receiver always has to be line-of-sight to the speaker's infrared transmitter (called an emitter). Therefore, if you turn away from the TV, or go to the kitchen, you won't hear anything until you return and face the TV again (line of sight remember). Anything or anybody coming between your infrared receiver and the emitter blocks the signal. I find these problems severely limit their usefulness, and I don't recommend them for that reason, but I've got nothing against the quality of their sound.

4. Induction Loop Systems

Induction loops are the most mysterious of the assistive devices because they use a varying magnetic field to transmit the sound from the assistive device to the t-coils in your hearing aids. These are among the cheapest and most versatile assistive devices available.

To use induction loops, you first need to have t-coils in your hearing aids. Induction loops "connect" to your hearing aids via their t-coils. There is no physical connection.

There are two "kinds" of induction loops. One is a neckloop (which you wear around your neck as the name implies) and plug it into whatever device you are listening to—whether a personal amplifier such as a PockeTalker, or an FM or infrared receiver, or directly into a radio or MP3 player or iPod. (Music Links are tiny devices that sit on your ears, but do the same job as neckloops.)

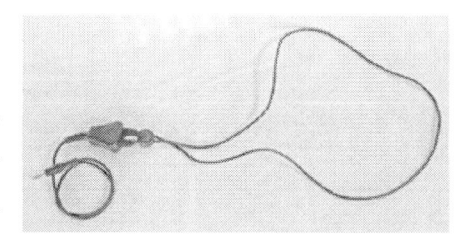

Neckloop

The other "kind" of induction loop is a room loop. The typical application for room loops is for meetings and for listening to the TV. If you install a room loop in your house, you can freely move around anywhere inside the loop and still hear the TV as well as you can sitting right in front of it. I have wired half of my house so I can move around anywhere in the living room, dining area and kitchen, or go downstairs, and still clearly hear my TV. Room loops are relatively inexpensive—under $200.00. They consist of a loop amplifier that is hooked to your TV (or other audio device), and a length of wire to circle the area you want looped.

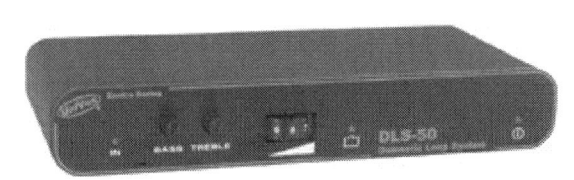

Univox DLS-50 Room Loop Amplifier

To learn more about loop systems and how they can help you, read my article, "Loop Systems—The Best-Kept Secret in Town!" (http://www.

hearinglosshelp.com/articles/loopsystems.htm). You can also see pictures and features of these loop amplifiers at http://www.hearinglosshelp.com/products/univoxdls50.htm.

5. Bluetooth Systems

The new kids on the block are systems that use bluetooth technology. Think of bluetooth as tiny built-in walkie-talkies that allow two devices to automatically "talk" to each other. The range of bluetooth is quite limited (a maximum of 30 feet, but 20 feet is a more reliable figure). With a bluetooth cell phone and a bluetooth device connected to your hearing aids (either directly attached, or via a bluetooth neckloop such as the CM-BT bluetooth neckloop, which you can get at http://www.hearinglosshelp.com/products/cmbt.htm), you can hear and talk on your cell phone even while it is in your purse or pocket. In addition to cell phones, you can use bluetooth to listen to any device that has bluetooth technology built in such as some computers, MP3 players, iPods, PDAs (personal digital assistants), etc.

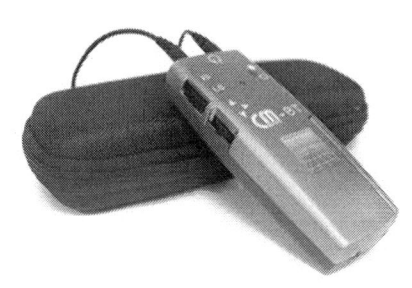

CM-BT Bluetooth Neckloop

Some higher end hearing aids such as the Oticon Epoq and the Phonak Exelia come with bluetooth technology built into their remote controls (streamers). You simply wear the "streamer" on a lanyard around your neck. The streamer receives the bluetooth signal from your cell phone, or other bluetooth device, and automatically re-transmits it to your hearing aids via its own proprietary technology.

Note that bluetooth devices need to be "paired" to each other before they will work. Thus several people cannot listen to one bluetooth device at the same time like they can with other technologies.

Amplified Telephones

While not a separate technology, many people have problems hearing on their phones. With phones, you can use several of the above technologies to help you hear better. For example, you can use your t-coils to "couple" with your phone's receiver. You can get special amplified phones that give you much more volume if that is your problem, or you can use a personal amplifier or in-line amplifier to boost your phone's volume. Some special phones have jacks in

Clarity XL50 Amplified Telephone

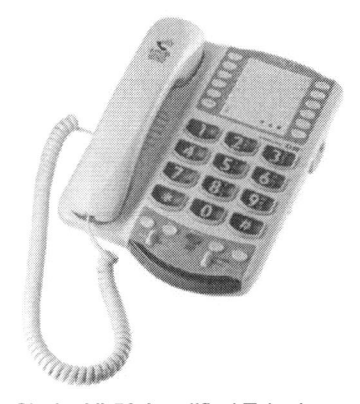

them so you can plug in a neckloop or direct audio input (DAI) patch cord. As well, many cell phones have bluetooth technology built in.

Pictured at the bottom of the previous page is one of the most powerful amplified phones currently made. It is the one I use and love. You can learn more about it at http://www.hearinglosshelp.com/products/clarityxl50.htm.

Connecting Your Hearing Aids to Assistive Devices

Typically, assistive devices can work with or without your hearing aids. However, most people choose to use them with their hearing aids. They want to know, "How do I make these wonderful assistive devices work with my hearing aids?"

Depending on your hearing aids, you may be able to couple assistive devices to your hearing aids by one or more of the following four basic methods.

T-coils

T-coils are sometimes called telecoils or audiocoils. The most common method of "connecting" assistive devices to your hearing aids is via their built-in t-coils. (Note: if you don't already have t-coils in your hearing aids, ask your audiologist if they can be retrofitted. I don't recommend buying hearing aids unless they have t-coils built in. They are that useful!)

If you are using a room loop, all you need to do is switch your hearing aids to their t-coil mode and hear beautiful clear sound (assuming you have the loop system hooked up and turned on). If you are using a personal loop such as a neckloop or the Music Links, you plug it into the earphone jack on the device you want to listen to. To learn more about t-coils and how useful they are, read my article called "Using T-Coils to Couple Your Hearing Aids to Various Audio Devices" available on the Center's website at http://www.hearinglosshelp.com/articles/tcoils.htm.

Direct Audio Input (DAI)

Some hearing aids and cochlear implants have a tiny jack on the hearing aid itself so you can plug in a "patch cord" and plug the other end directly into the device to which you want to listen—e. g. a radio, iPod, MP3 player, computer or various FM receivers and personal amplifiers. Unfortunately, few hearing aids today have DAI jacks or "boots".

Some higher end hearing aids such as the Oticon Epoq and the Phonak Exelia have direct audio input jacks built into their remote controls (streamers). You simply wear the "streamer" on a lanyard around your neck. It receives the sound signal from the device you have plugged your patch cord into and automatically re-transmits it to your hearing aids via its own proprietary technology.

FM receivers

A few hearing aids have built-in FM receivers, or have special "boots" so you can attach a tiny FM receiver to them. You then listen to the speaker via the corresponding wireless FM microphone he wears. The downside is that these tiny systems are expensive and limit you to certain brands of hearing aids. Also, if you get new hearing aids, you need to get new FM receivers and that just adds to the expense. (Much better, in my opinion, although bigger and clunkier, is to get a separate FM receiver and listen to it via a neckloop. That way it can work with any hearing aid, or even without any hearing aid.)

Bluetooth

Bluetooth technology is similar to the tiny FM receivers (above), but bluetooth receivers are limited to a distance of under 30 feet (really only effective to about 20 feet). With bluetooth you can listen to bluetooth-enabled devices without any wires connecting to your hearing aids.

In the past, assistive devices have been one of the best kept secrets in town. Few hard of hearing people were aware of their existence, and even fewer knew where to purchase them. Fortunately, that is no longer true. Now you know about assistive devices too. You have learned just how useful they can be. When used with your hearing aids in difficult listening situations, the two make an awesome combination! If you want to learn more about these wonderful devices, you can find all kinds of them on the Center's website at http://www.hearinglosshelp.com/products.htm.

The Last Word

You have now learned the six "Keys to Successfully Living with Your Hearing Loss". As you apply each of these six keys to your life, you will soon realize just how much more confident and happier you are because you can now hear and understand much of what people say. You have rejoined the hearing world on your own terms. Its great, isn't it?

Good Books on Hearing Loss

Integrity First Books in the series:

Everything You Wanted to Know About Your Hearing Loss But Were Afraid to Ask
(Because You Knew You Wouldn't Hear the Answers Anyway!)
by Neil G. Bauman, Ph.D.

If you have enjoyed this book and would like to learn more about hearing loss and how you can successfully live with it, you may be interested in some helpful books by Dr. Neil. Each book is packed with the things you need to know in order to thrive in spite of your various hearing loss issues. The direct link to the following books is at www.hearinglosshelp.com/products/books.htm.

Ototoxic Drugs Exposed—The Shocking Truth About Prescription Drugs, Medications, Chemicals and Herbals That Can (and Do) Damage Our Ears ($52.45; eBook $39.95)

This book, now in its third edition, reveals the shocking truth that many prescription drugs can damage your ears. Some drugs slowly and insidiously rob you of your hearing, cause your ears to ring or destroy your balance. Other drugs can smash your ears in one fell swoop, leaving you with profound, permanent hearing loss and bringing traumatic change into your life. Learn how to protect your ears from the ravages of ototoxic drugs and chemicals. Describes the specific ototoxic effects of 877 drugs, 35 herbals and 148 chemicals (798 pages).

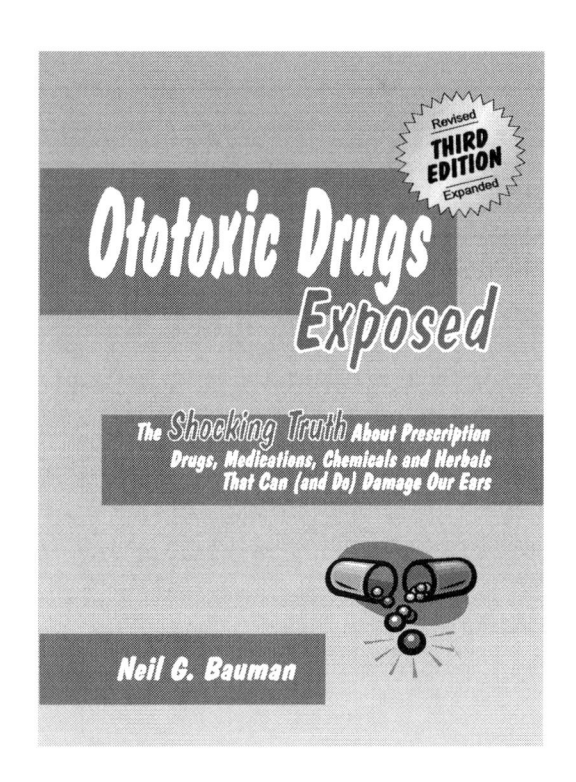

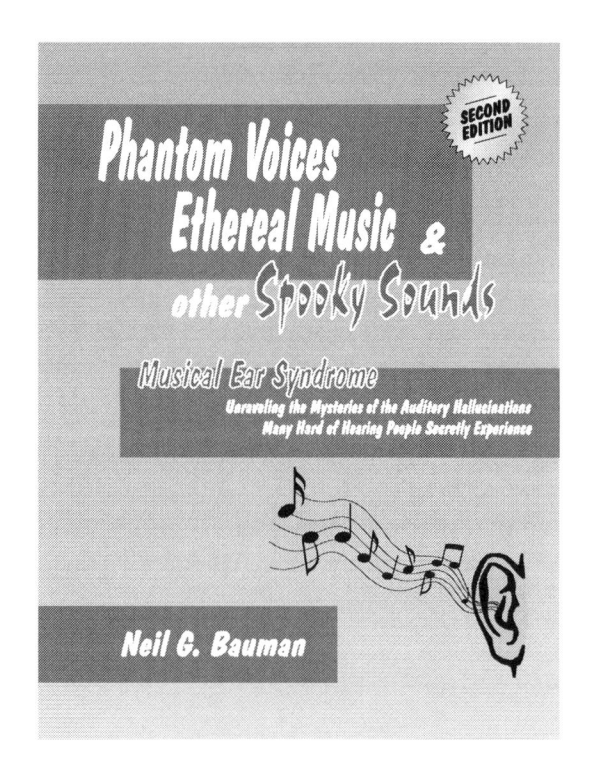

Phantom Voices, Ethereal Music & Other Spooky Sounds ($22.49; eBook $16.99)

When you realize you are hearing phantom sounds, you immediately think that something has gone dreadfully wrong "upstairs"—that you are going crazy. Because of this, few people openly talk about the strange phantom voices, music, singing and other spooky sounds they hear. This book, the first of its kind in the world, lifts the veil on "Musical Ear syndrome" and reveals numerous first-hand accounts of the many strange phantom sounds people experience. Not only that, it explains what causes these phantom sounds, and more importantly, what you can do to eliminate them, or at least, bring them under control (164 pages).

When Your Ears Ring! Cope with Your Tinnitus—Here's How ($18.95; eBook $14.49)

If your ears ring, buzz, chirp, hiss or roar, you know just how annoying tinnitus can be. You do not have to put up with this racket for the rest of your life. Recent studies show that a lot of what we thought we knew about tinnitus is not true at all. Exciting new research reveals what you can do to eliminate or greatly reduce the severity of your tinnitus. In this book you will learn what causes tinnitus in the first place and the steps you can take to bring it under control (118 pages).

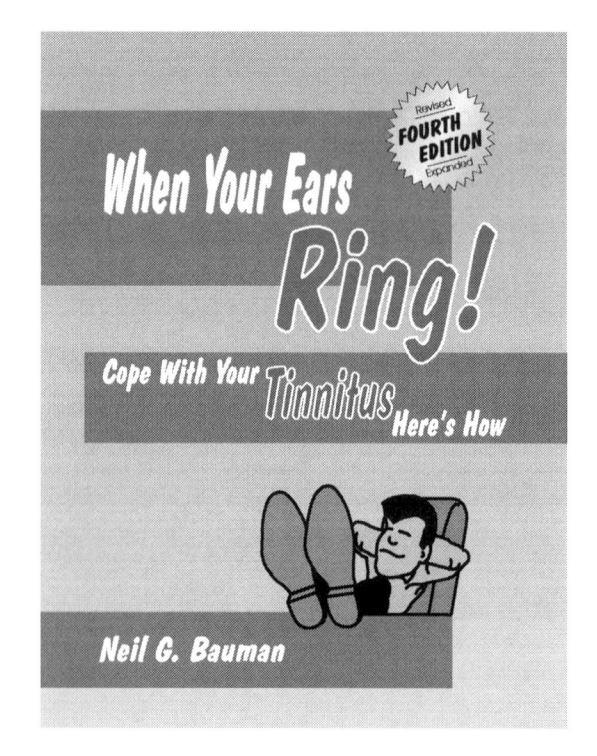

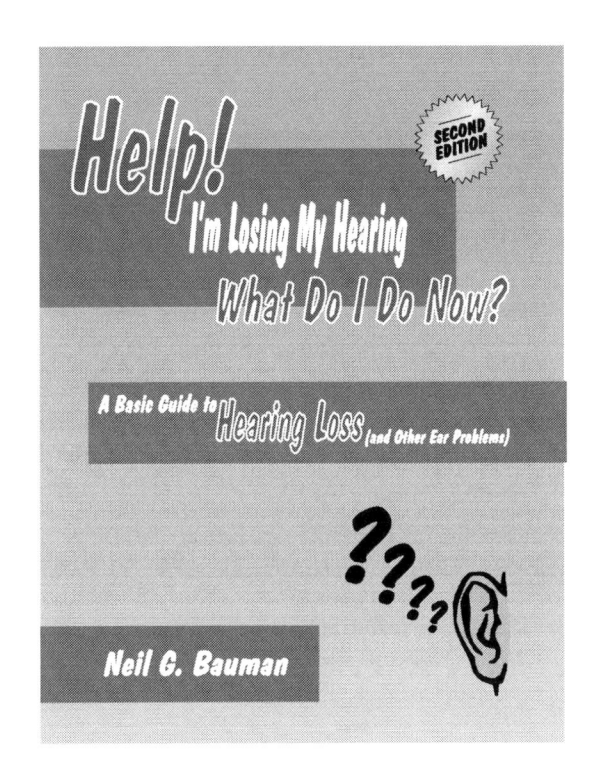

Help! I'm Losing My Hearing—What Do I Do Now? ($18.95; eBook $14.49)

Losing your hearing can flip your world upside down and leave your mind in a turmoil. You may be full of fears, wondering how you will be able to live the rest of your life as a hard of hearing person. You don't know where to turn. You lament, "What do I do now?" Set your mind at rest. This easy to read book, written by a fellow hard of hearing person, is packed with the information and resources you need to successfully deal with your hearing loss and other ear conditions. (118 pages).

Keys to Successfully Living with Your Hearing Loss ($19.97; eBook $15.49)

Do you know: a) the critical missing element to successfully living with your hearing loss? b) that the No. 1 coping strategy hard of hearing people instinctively use is wrong, wrong, wrong? c) what the single most effective hearing loss coping strategy is? d) how you can turn your hearing aids into awesome hearing devices? This book addresses the surprising answers to these and other critical questions. Applying them to your life will put you well on the road to successfully living with your hearing loss. (84 pages).

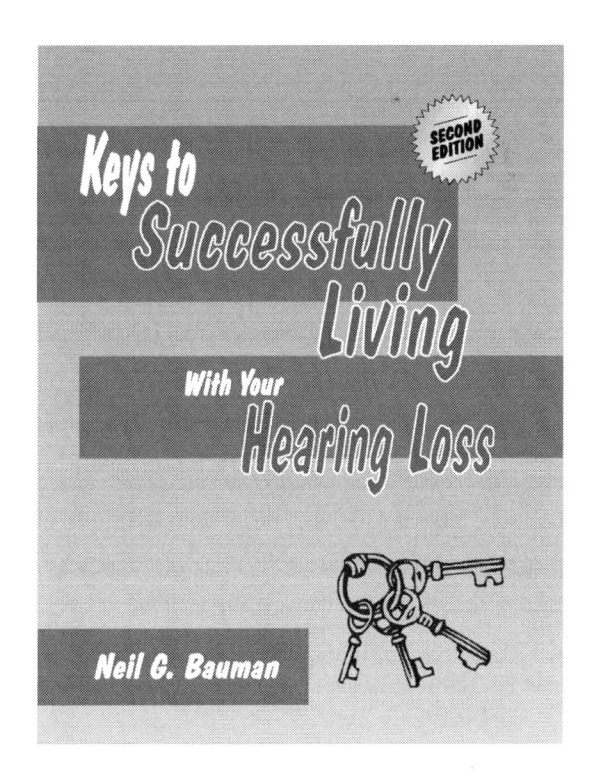

The Agony of Meniere's Disease—Please Make My World Stop Spinning ($18.95; eBook $14.49)

Meniere's Disease is one of the more incapacitating things you can experience. If you suffer from your world spinning and have a fluctuating hearing loss together with noises in your ears, this book is for you. It explains what is known about Meniere's, its causes and the best treatments available today. There are lots of hints that you can try out for yourself to reduce or eliminate the effects of Meniere's disease. Since everyone is different, see what works for you (80 pages).

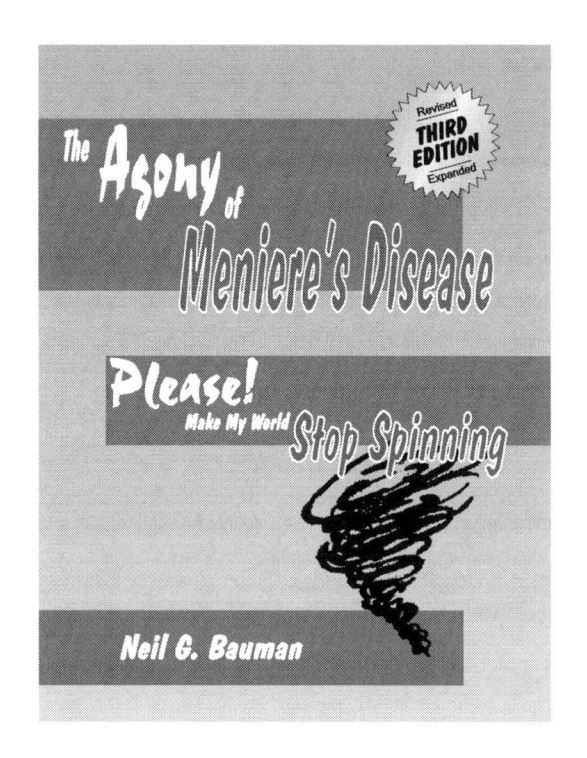

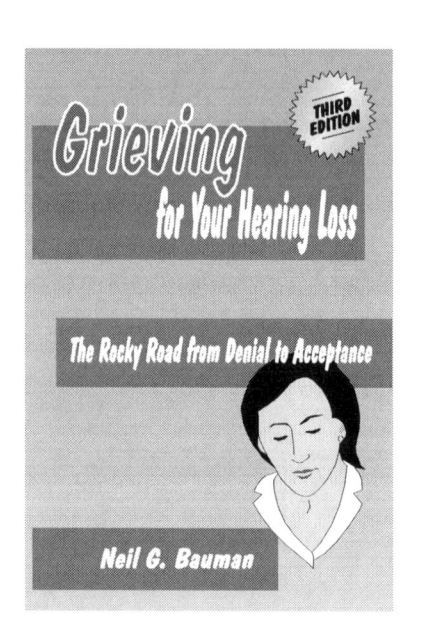

Grieving for Your Hearing Loss—The Rocky Road from Denial to Acceptance ($12.95; eBook $9.95)

When you lose your hearing you need to grieve. This is not optional—but critical to your continued mental and physical health. This book leads you through the process of dealing with the grief and pain you experience as a result of your hearing loss. It explains what you are going through each step of the way. It gives you hope when you are in the depths of despair and depression. It shows you how you can lead a happy vibrant life again in spite of your hearing loss. This book has helped many (56 pages).

Good Books on Hearing Loss

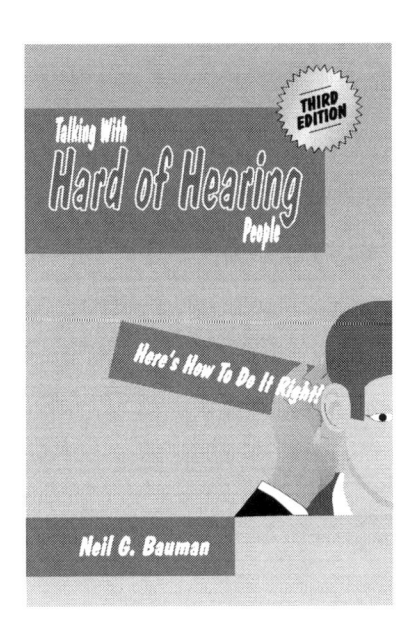

Talking with Hard of Hearing People—Here's How to Do It Right! ($9.95; eBook $7.95)

Talking is important to all of us. When communication breaks down, we all suffer. For hard of hearing people this happens all the time. This book is for you—whether you are hearing or hard of hearing! It explains how to communicate with hard of hearing people in one-to-one situations, in groups and meetings, in emergency situations, and in hospitals and nursing homes. When you use the principles given in this book, good things will happen and you will finally be able to have a comfortable chat with a hard of hearing person (38 pages).

When Hearing Loss Ambushes Your Ears—Here's What Happens When Your Hearing Goes on the Fritz ($14.95; eBook $11.95)

Hearing loss often blindsides you. As a result, your first step should be to learn as much as you can about your hearing loss; then you will be able to cope better. This most interesting book explains how your ears work, the causes of hearing loss, what you can expect to hear with different levels of hearing loss and why you often can't understand what you hear. Lots of audiograms and charts help make things clear. You will also discover a lot of fascinating things about how loud noises damage your ears (88 pages).

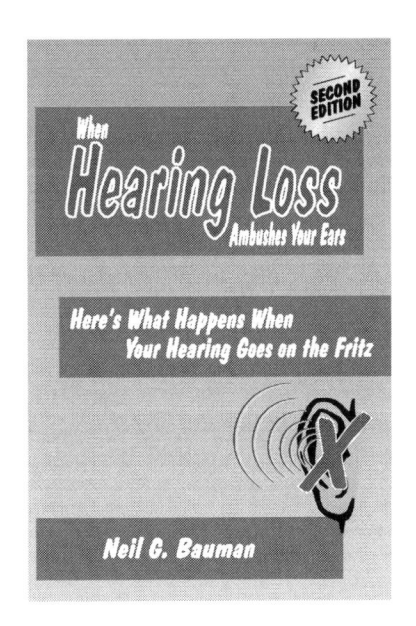

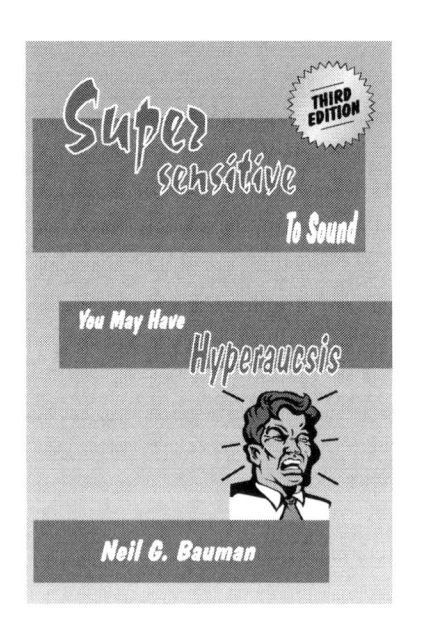

Supersensitive to Sound? You May Have Hyperacusis ($9.95; eBook $7.95)

If some (or all) normal sounds seem so loud they blow your socks off, this is the book you want to read! You don't have to avoid noise or lock yourself away in a soundproof room. Exciting new research on this previously baffling problem reveals what you can do to help bring your hyperacusis under control (42 pages).

Here! Here! You and Your Hearing Loss/You and Your Hearing Aids ($12.95; eBook $10.95)

Part I of this book contains a series of my newspaper articles on hearing loss such as, "Hear Today. Gone Tomorrow?" "Hearing Loss Is Sneaky!" "The Wages of Din Is Deaf!" "When Your Ears Ring..." "Get In My Face Before You Speak!" "How's That Again?" "Being Hard of Hearing Is Hard" "I'm Deaf, Not Daft!" Part II contains articles on hearing aids such as, "You Better Watch Out..." "Before Buying Your First Hearing Aid..." "Please Don't Lock Me Away in Your Drawer" "Good-bye World of Silence!" "Becoming Friends with Your Hearing Aids" "Two's Better Than One!" (56 pages).

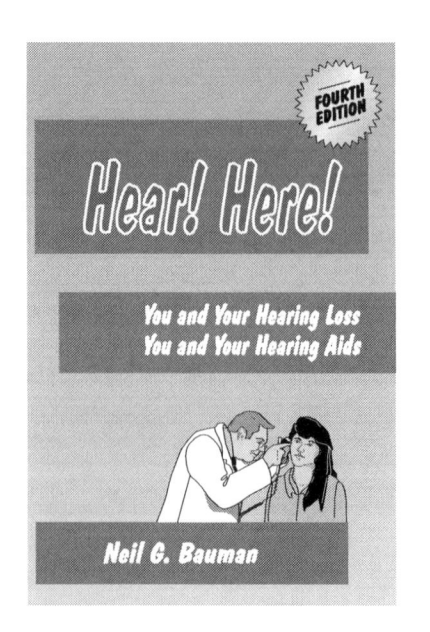

You can order any of the foregoing books/eBooks (plus you can read more than 500 other helpful articles about hearing loss and related issues) from the
Center for Hearing Loss Help
web site at
http://www.hearinglosshelp.com
or order them from the address below

Center for Hearing Loss Help

49 Piston Court,
Stewartstown, PA 17363-8322
Phone: (717) 993-8555
FAX: (717) 993-6661
E-mail: info@hearinglosshelp.com
Web site: http://www.hearinglosshelp.com

Made in the USA
Charleston, SC
06 June 2012